Bariatric Air Fryer Cookbook

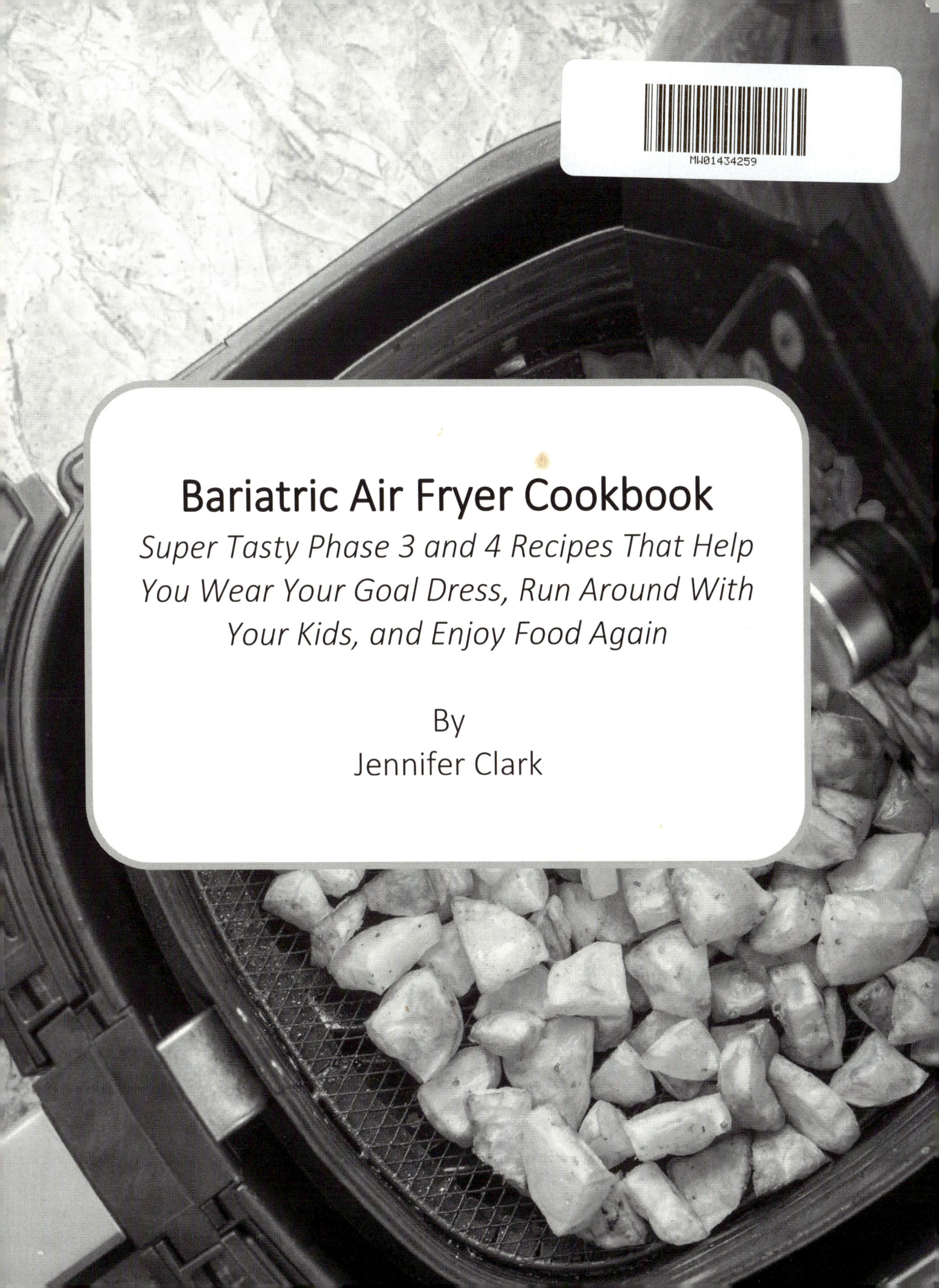

Super Tasty Phase 3 and 4 Recipes That Help You Wear Your Goal Dress, Run Around With Your Kids, and Enjoy Food Again

By
Jennifer Clark

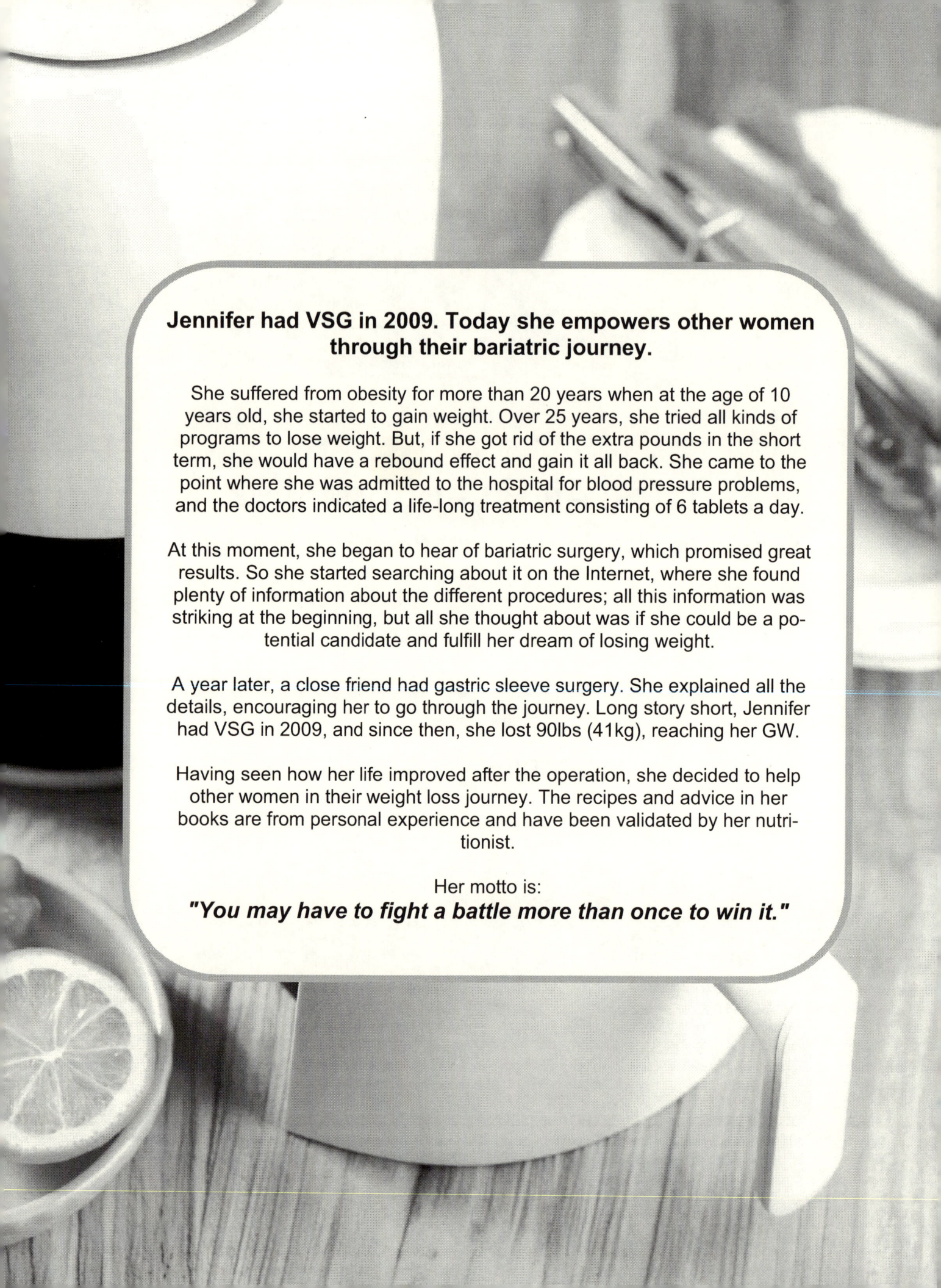

Jennifer had VSG in 2009. Today she empowers other women through their bariatric journey.

She suffered from obesity for more than 20 years when at the age of 10 years old, she started to gain weight. Over 25 years, she tried all kinds of programs to lose weight. But, if she got rid of the extra pounds in the short term, she would have a rebound effect and gain it all back. She came to the point where she was admitted to the hospital for blood pressure problems, and the doctors indicated a life-long treatment consisting of 6 tablets a day.

At this moment, she began to hear of bariatric surgery, which promised great results. So she started searching about it on the Internet, where she found plenty of information about the different procedures; all this information was striking at the beginning, but all she thought about was if she could be a potential candidate and fulfill her dream of losing weight.

A year later, a close friend had gastric sleeve surgery. She explained all the details, encouraging her to go through the journey. Long story short, Jennifer had VSG in 2009, and since then, she lost 90lbs (41kg), reaching her GW.

Having seen how her life improved after the operation, she decided to help other women in their weight loss journey. The recipes and advice in her books are from personal experience and have been validated by her nutritionist.

Her motto is:
"You may have to fight a battle more than once to win it."

CONTENTS

The Best Kitchen Tool For Post-Op 7
Empowering Eating Habits For Phases 3 And 4 8
Faq: You Ask And I Answer 9
Tips & Tricks For A Perfect Frying 10
Conversion Charts 11

BREAKFAST 13

Almond And Blueberry Muffins 14
Almond Donuts 14
Apple Cake 15
Apple Treats 15
Banana And Chocolate Brownies 16
Banana Bread 16
Banana Chips 17
Banana Split 17
Berry Tacos 18
Butter Cookies 18
Cheesecake Treats 19
Chocolate Balls 19
Chocolate Cake 20
Chocolate Chip Cookies 20
Chocolate Cream 21
Chocolate Cups 21
Chocolate Pudding 21
Cinnamon Toast 22
Cocoa And Almond Bars 22
Coffee Cake 22
Cookie Doughnuts 23
Crispy Apple Chips 23
Fried Bananas 24
Fried Peaches 24
Orange Cookies 25
Peanut Butter And Jelly Doughnuts 25
Pineapple Sweets 26
Plum And Currant Cake 26
Poached Apples 27

Pumpkin Cookies 27
Simple Cookies 28
Snow-White Cake 28
Sweet Potato Croquettes 29
Vanilla Blueberry Muffins 29

LUNCH 31

Beef In Red Wine Reduction 32
Beef Tenderloin With Butter 32
Breaded Sole 33
Broccoli And Cheese Croquettes 33
Broccoli And Mushroom Omelet 34
Broccoli And Tofu Risotto 34
Butter Fried Chicken 35
Butter Salmon 35
Cauliflower & Cheese 35
Chicken Breast 36
Chicken Fajita With Spicy Potatoes 36
Chicken Wings 37
Cordon Bleu 37
Creamy Salmon 38
Fish And Chips 38
Fried Chicken Fillets 38
Garlic And Spice Chicken Burger 39
Garlic Pork Tenderloins 39
Ham And Bell Pepper Omelet 39
Hamburger And Tzatziki 40
Kebab 40
Lamb Burger 40
Meatloaf 41
Minced Meat 41
Mozzarella Schnitzel 41
Mushroom, Beef, And Leek Pie 42
Oregano Clams 42
Paprika And Lemon Grilled Chicken 43
Porcini Mushroom Stake 43

Pork Ribs 44
Roast Beef 44
Sausage And Vegetable Sandwich 44
Seasoned Cod Fillets 45
Spicy Hamburger 45
Tasty Salmon 45
Tofu With Vegetables 46
Turkey And Avocado Burger 46
Turkey Wings 46
Vegetarian Toast 47
White Wine Chicken Breast 47

DINNER 49
"Chipotle" Steaks 50
Beef And Beans 50
Beef Kebab 50
Beef Tacos 51
Calamari Skewers In Vermouth 51
Cauliflower Balls 52
Cheese Pork Chops 52
Chicken Slices With Peppers 52
Classic Schnitzel 53
Coconut-Flavored Brussels Sprouts 53
Cod Fillets With Parmesan Cheese 53
Fish Tacos 54
Flounder Fillets With Parmesan Cheese 54
Fried Sardines 55
Garlic Calamari 55
German-Style Schnitzel 55
Gnocchi With Parmesan Cheese And Cauliflower 56
Italian-Style Pork Tenderloins 56
Lamb Chops 57
Lemon Lamb Steaks 57
Meatballs 57
Mozzarella Crostone With Chicken And Peppers 58
Oriental-Style Spiced Lamb 58
Paprika Bacon Cubes 58
Paprika Pork Ribs 59

Parmesan Trout 59
Plain Steak 60
Pork Chops With 4 Kinds Of Cheese 60
Pork Ribs With Parmesan Cheese 60
Salmon Fillets In Walnut Crust 61
Trout With Garlic And Lemon 61
Sesame Pork Ribs 62
Smoked Steaks 62
Spice Marinated Chicken 63
Spiced Pork Steaks 63
Sweet-And-Sour Pork Steaks 64
Thyme And Mushrooms Meatloaf 64
Tuna Steak With Red Onions 65
Turmeric-Orange Marinated Steak 65
Western-Style Pork Loin 65

VEGETABLES AND SALADS 67
Avocado Eggs 68
Bell Pepper Salad 68
Corn And Tomato Salad 68
Creamy Zucchini And Potatoes 69
Crispy Broccoli Salad 69
Crunchy Green Beans 69
Eggs And Tomatoes 70
Herb Lentils 70
Leek Salad 70
Oregano Peppers 71
Oriental-Style Asparagus 71
Spinach Salad 71
Zucchini Salad 72

SNACKS 73
Almond Sandwiches 74
Avocado Sticks 74
Bacon-Wrapped Avocado 75
Blueberry Pudding 75
Breaded Zucchini Chips 76

Brussels Sprouts With Thyme And Parsley 76
Calamari Rings With Almonds 76
Cauliflower And Cheese Gnocchi 77
Cheese And Bacon Broccoli 77
Cheese Fried Zucchini 78
Cheese Sticks 78
Cheese Cauliflower 78
Cinnamon Cupcakes 79
Classic Frankfurters 79
Coconut And Vanilla Treats 79
Cucumber And Mozzarella Wrap 80
Greek-Style Eggs 80
Healthy Fries 81
Herb Crab Cake 81
Lemon Pie 82
Lentils And Dates Brownies 82
Melted Cheese Cups 83
Mexican-Style Cheese Sticks 83
Mozzarella Cheese Cubes And Paprika 83
Puerto Rican-Style Banana 84
Roasted Nut Mix 84
Seaweed Chips 84
Sesame-Seasoned Broccoli 85
Soft Cake 85
Spicy Bacon Bites 86
Strawberry Sweets 86
Taco Chips 87
Tangerine Pudding 87
Zucchini Chips 87

DESSERTS 89
Air Fried Biscuits 90
Almond Cookies 90
Almonds And Peanut Butter Balls 91
Apple And Raisin Pastries 91
Apple Chips 92
Apple Cinnamon Pie 92
Apple Pastries 93
Apple Rolls 93
Apple-Flavored Bites 94
Butter And Stevia Pie 94
Cake Bites 94
Caramel And Coconut Cream 95
Cherry Pie 95
Chocolate And Peanut Butter Cookies 96
Chocolate Cupcake With Chocolate Cream 96
Chocolate Mug Cake 97
Chocolate Sufflè 97
Cinnamon Pear Chips 97
Coconut And Honey Apricots 98
Currant And Chocolate Cupcakes 98
Danish Cinnamon Rolls 98
Deep-Fried Bananas With Chocolate Sauce 99
Easy Biscuits 99
Fried Cinnamon Bananas 100
Fried Plantains 100
Hazelnut Cake 100
Lemon Butter Cookies 101
Peanut Butter And Marshmallow Croissants 101
Pineapple Yogurt Sticks 102
Rum Pancakes 102
Strawberry Shortcakes 103
Vanilla Cookies 103
Vanilla-Cinnamon Cookies 103
Vanilla Mug Cake 104

BONUS GUIDES 105
Tips And Tricks To Prevent Hair Loss 106
How To Overcome Stalls 107
Conclusion 109
Shopping List 110
Index 111

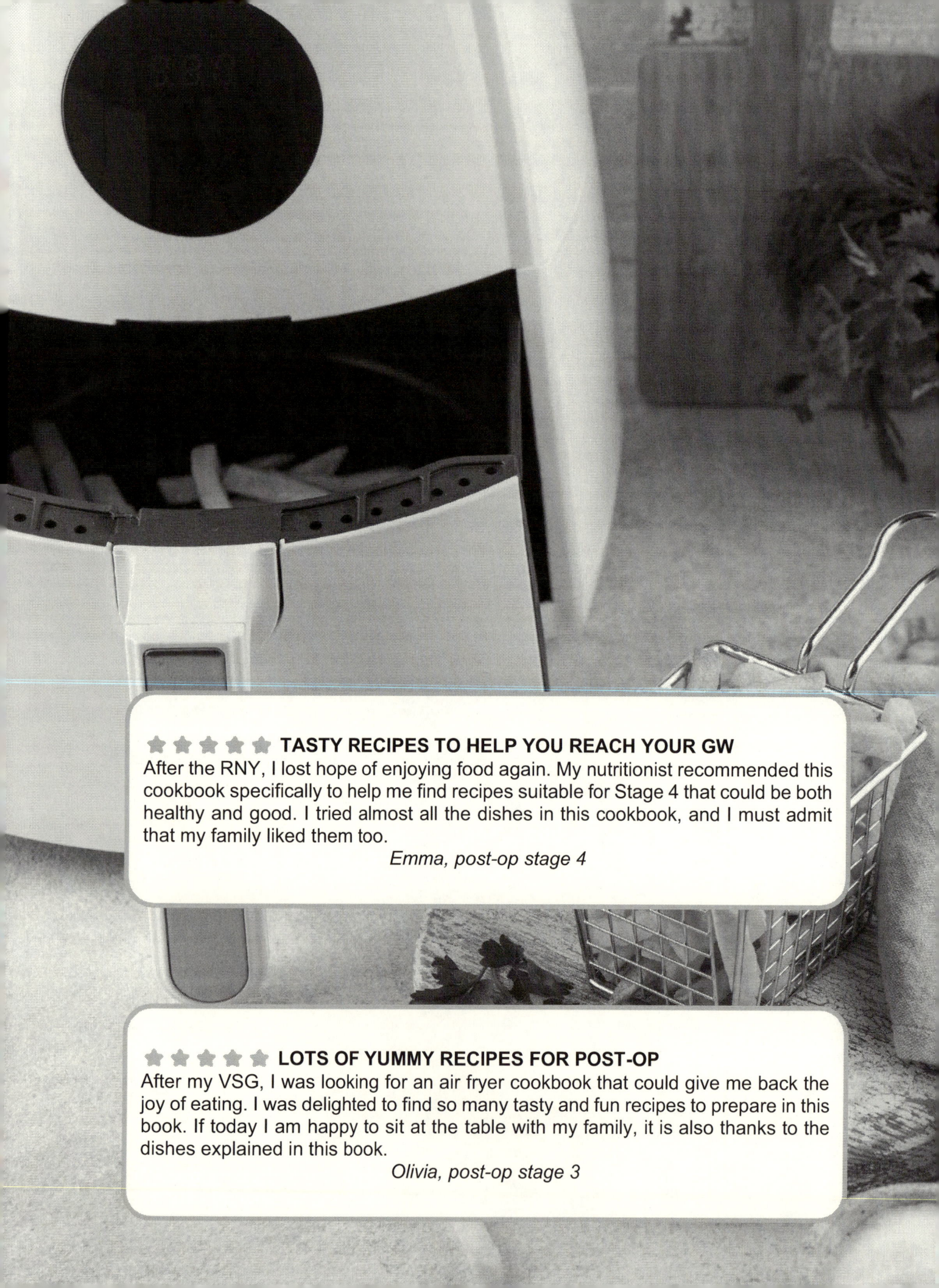

⭐⭐⭐⭐⭐ **TASTY RECIPES TO HELP YOU REACH YOUR GW**
After the RNY, I lost hope of enjoying food again. My nutritionist recommended this cookbook specifically to help me find recipes suitable for Stage 4 that could be both healthy and good. I tried almost all the dishes in this cookbook, and I must admit that my family liked them too.

Emma, post-op stage 4

⭐⭐⭐⭐⭐ **LOTS OF YUMMY RECIPES FOR POST-OP**
After my VSG, I was looking for an air fryer cookbook that could give me back the joy of eating. I was delighted to find so many tasty and fun recipes to prepare in this book. If today I am happy to sit at the table with my family, it is also thanks to the dishes explained in this book.

Olivia, post-op stage 3

THE BEST KITCHEN TOOL FOR POST-OP

Hi, I'm Jennifer, and as you may have guessed, I'm the author of this book. If you want to get straight to the action, then go to page 12, where you will find the first recipes. If, on the other hand, you are curious to learn more about the air fryer and how it can help you in your bariatric journey, then keep reading.

The tool that is changing the way bariatric surgery patients cook

The air fryer has become the most popular cooking tool over the last few years among bariatric surgery patients. The increased focus on proper nutrition after surgery and the demand for "real food taste" have allowed this product to become commonplace among those who laid on the loser's bench.

An eye on your weight...

The air fryer uses hot air between 150 and 200 degrees instead of oil to fry food. This makes it possible to cook variations of traditionally fried dishes, with the same taste but with far fewer calories and fats, which makes them perfect for those following the post-op bariatric diet.

Unlike other cooking methods, the air fryer does not use radiation or microwaves to cook food. Instead, it relies on a heat source, similar to what can be found in convection ovens, which causes hot air to flow around the food. It is this circulation of hot air that allows for cooking similar to that of a standard deep fryer without extra calories.

...and one on the taste

The air fryer is truly unique because it allows you to replicate the taste of your favorite foods you have not been able to eat for quite some time. This makes it a great companion for anyone in stages 3 and 4, who can finally reintroduce solid foods after months of liquids.

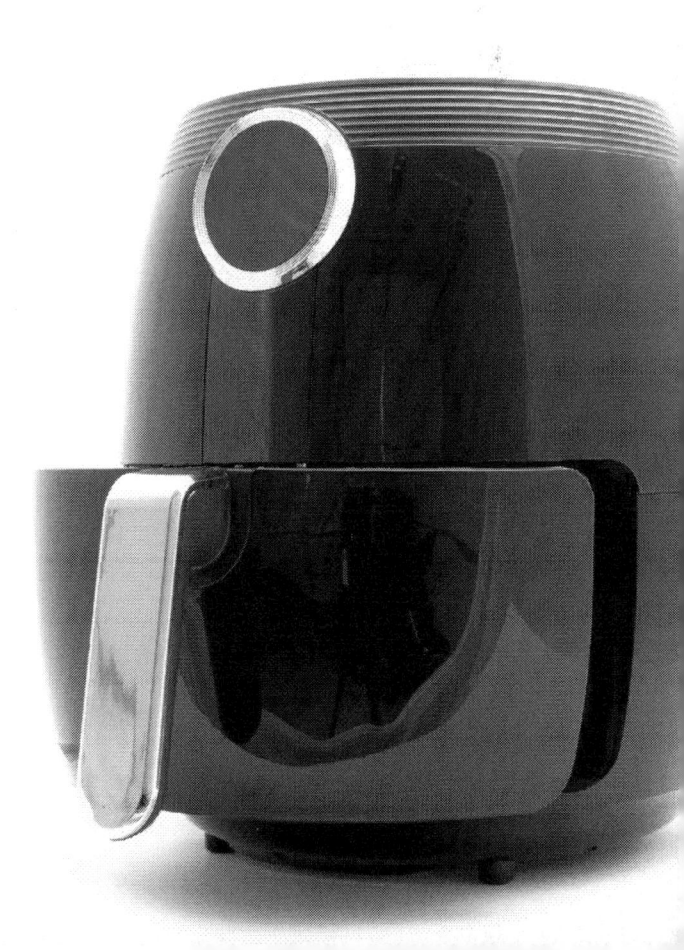

EMPOWERING EATING HABITS FOR PHASES 3 AND 4

When entering phase 3 and then phase 4, it is essential to start developing eating habits that can sustain weight loss over the long term. It is not uncommon for patients undergoing bariatric surgery to regain the weight they lost within a year of the operation. To ensure that this does not happen and to be able to enjoy food again, here are the tips that helped me along the way.

Rest the cutlery on the plate after each bite
This is a trick to lengthen the duration of the meal, making us feel like we are eating more than we have on the plate. Nothing is more stressful than finishing one's portion when others have just started eating. Since the amount of food we can consume is quite limited, letting some time pass between bites allows us to keep up with others. Try it to believe it.

Drink only outside of meals
Reducing the size of the stomach results in it filling up faster. Water, as well as any other liquid, contributes to the feeling of fullness. While this can be good during the pre-op diet, after bariatric surgery, it becomes essential to be able to consume the calories prescribed by the nutritionist. In this sense, feeling full before you have completed your meal can lead to too low a caloric intake, which causes slowdowns in metabolism and does not allow you to have the strength you need to live normally. In addition, drinking outside of meals ensures that you have the space to enjoy the meal until the last bite.

Chew each bite well and savor it to the fullest
Bariatric surgery can also be an opportunity to rediscover flavors we took for granted. Chewing for at least 20 seconds with each bite not only lengthens the time of the meal but also eases digestion and allows us to savor every nuance of what we are eating. And trust me, the recipes in this book are worth enjoying to the fullest.

Replace sugar with less caloric variants
Sugar makes everything taste better, and there is no doubt about that. Unfortunately, however, this food is certainly not a good companion for those who have undergone bariatric surgery. Sugar has a high caloric density that is likely to easily overshoot the daily intake indicated by the nutritionist. Fortunately for us, natural variants, such as liquid stevia, achieve the same flavor but with a hundredth of the calories of sugar. In the recipes in this book, you will find only natural sweeteners readily available in the supermarket.

Proteins are key
Protein is one of the best allies of those who have had bariatric surgery. They perform many valuable functions, including building and maintaining muscle mass. In addition, favoring protein-rich dishes during stages 3 and 4 allows you to reduce loose skin and avoid hair loss, which is often an object of anxiety and concern for women.

Eat very slowly
To avoid dumping syndrome, eating slowly is essential. To go into more detail, I recommend taking at least 30 minutes per meal and 60 minutes to drink one cup of water.

If you follow these steps carefully and make them into actual habits, I am sure you will soon be back to enjoying your favorite dishes in serenity. And at that point, fitting into your goal dress will be a breeze!

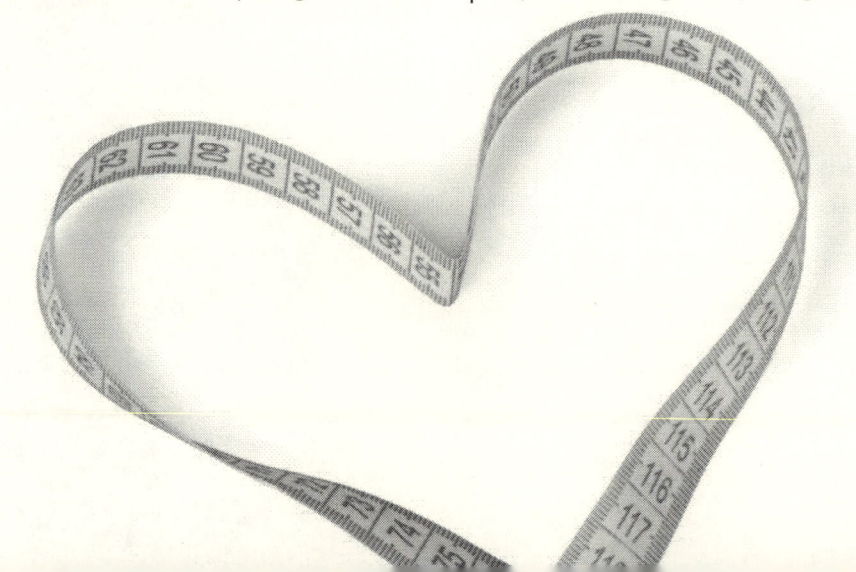

FAQ: YOU ASK AND I ANSWER

Beginners may have seemingly trivial questions about cooking with an air fryer. Don't worry, I'm here to provide the answer to your doubts.

Can baking paper be used in the air fryer?
Of course, but be sure to poke holes in it so that air can circulate freely. Otherwise, you risk the food not cooking as it should.

What about tinfoil?
The same argument made for baking paper applies. I generally recommend using it only in recipes that specifically require it.

I have a silicone baking pan. Can I use it in the air fryer?
Absolutely. There are no contraindications. Just make sure it can withstand the high temperatures of the air fryer.

I just bought an air fryer. Can I start cooking or are there steps I need to do first?
I recommend that you stick to your air fryer's instruction booklet. If by now you have read dozens of sites that have convinced you that there will be an unpleasant plastic smell the first few times and you want to do something to prevent this, you can dilute some apple cider vinegar in a glass of water and run it at 350F for 10 minutes.

Can I cook frozen foods directly from the freezer?
Yes. There is no need to thaw them beforehand.

I was told that it is always better to add a little oil. Is this true?
That is an urban legend! In an air fryer, oil should only be used for recipes that explicitly call for it. Otherwise, there is no need to get your hands dirty. If you fear that the food you are about to cook may stick to the bottom of the air fryer, you can use an oil spray to grease the base and prevent this from happening.

Do I have to preheat the fryer before using it?
This is not mandatory. In some recipes, it is recommended, but there are no contraindications in cooking food without preheating the air fryer first. This is because, being fairly small, it takes a short time to reach the temperature. Furthermore, not preheating the fryer also saves you even more money.

Are there any special accessories I need to buy?
No, you can use the tools you already have at home. As for pans, molds, and cake pans, just make sure they can withstand high temperatures before you use them. If you don't, you may find yourself with some unpleasant surprises.

Can it be dangerous to run the air fryer near other appliances?
It is not dangerous, but it is always good to place it at least 1 foot from walls, electrical outlets, and utensils.

Can I put my air fryer in the dishwasher?
It depends on the model, but most newer ones can be washed in the dishwasher. Of course, I am referring exclusively to the basket and its container.

It says I cannot wash it in the dishwasher. Can I use a metal sponge?
No. Use a soft sponge instead. The bottom of the basket and its container are lined with a nonstick material, which would be scratched if washed with tools that are too hard on them.

How often should I wash the air fryer?
To avoid the formation of bad odors, I recommend that you clean it after each use.

Can I leave the power cord plugged in even when I am not using the fryer?
If this happens, it is not a problem. However, I recommend that you unplug it when you are not using it.

Are there any foods that cannot be cooked with the air fryer?
In theory, no. In practice, I advise against any food that you would not consume cooked in a classic oven.

TIPS & TRICKS FOR A PERFECT FRYING

Despite being an easy-to-use tool, the proper use of the air fryer remains a mystery to this day for many of its owners. Don't worry, in this chapter I list the most common mistakes and how to avoid them to ensure perfect frying.

Overfilling the fryer
This is a classic of first-timers. Overloading the air fryer is never a smart idea. Remember that the air fryer cooks food by circulating hot air. If you fill it up like a turkey, you can't expect much cooking. My advice is to spread the foods out by overlapping them as little as possible.

Forgetting to stir while cooking
Just as you need the air fryer to enjoy the goodness of fried food and stay in shape, she needs your help to function at her best. By stirring often you allow the food to cook evenly. Don't worry, I will remind you in most recipes to do this.

Using too much oil
Raise your hand if you have spent hundreds of dollars on an air fryer but consume a bottle of oil every two weeks because in your opinion "it tastes better that way." Okay, you can put your hand down. The truth is that too much oil can have the opposite effect and damage the fryer. Stick to the amount given in the recipes. Remember: perfect frying doesn't need that much oil.

Not using oil at all
Wait, you just told me that too much oil is not good and now you tell me that not using it at all is also a problem? Aurea Mediocritas said Horace: The truth lies in the middle. Oil remains an excellent vehicle to transfer heat, and the right dosage helps make food crispier. Stick to the amounts given in the recipes and you'll be good.

Frying moist or even wet foods
If food comes out of your air fryer having the consistency of a bath sponge, it is because you did not dry it before cooking it. As a result, the liquid evaporated during cooking, creating a moist environment. A paper towel roll is an essential companion for anyone who cooks with an air fryer. You will be pointed out in the recipes when it is best to dry foods before cooking them; do not worry: you are in good hands.

Cutting foods into pieces that are too small
Remember that the basket of the air fryer is perforated at the bottom to allow hot air to circulate. If you cut food into pieces that are too small, they may fall on the heating source. The result? Smoke all over the place and a recipe to redo. Over time you'll get the eye of how small is too small; when in doubt, it is better to use slightly larger pieces.

Not all fats are created equal
If you cook particularly fatty foods, the fat will drip to the bottom during cooking. The difference between a happy family meal and a ruined Sunday is what the fat will drip on. If it drips on the metal of the basket, then it will burn and the result will be a nice charred dish; if, on the other hand, it drips on water, put there especially for this eventuality, you can serve a mouth-watering meal. Your choice.

DRY WEIGHTS

OZ	Spoons	Cups	Grams
½ oz	1 tbsp	-	15g
1 oz	2 tbsp	1/8 c	28g
2 oz	4 tbsp	1/4 c	57g
3 oz	6 tbsp	1/3 c	85g
4 oz	8 tbsp	1/2 c	115g
8 oz	16 tbsp	1 c	227g
12 oz	24 tbsp	1 ½ c	340g
16 oz	32 tbsp	2 c	455g

LIQUID VOLUMES

OZ	Spoons	Cups	Ml
1 oz	2 tbsp	1/8 c	30 ml
2 oz	4 tbsp	1/4 c	60 ml
2 2/3 oz	6 tbsp	1/3 c	80 ml
4 oz	8 tbsp	1/2 c	120 ml
8 oz	16 tbsp	2/3 c	160 ml
12 oz	24 tbsp	3/4 c	177 ml
16 oz	32 tbsp	1 c	237 ml
32 oz	64 tbsp	1 ½ c	470 ml
		2 c	950 ml

TEMPERATURE

130 c	250 F
165 c	325 F
177 c	350 F
190 c	375 F
200 c	400 F
220 c	425 F

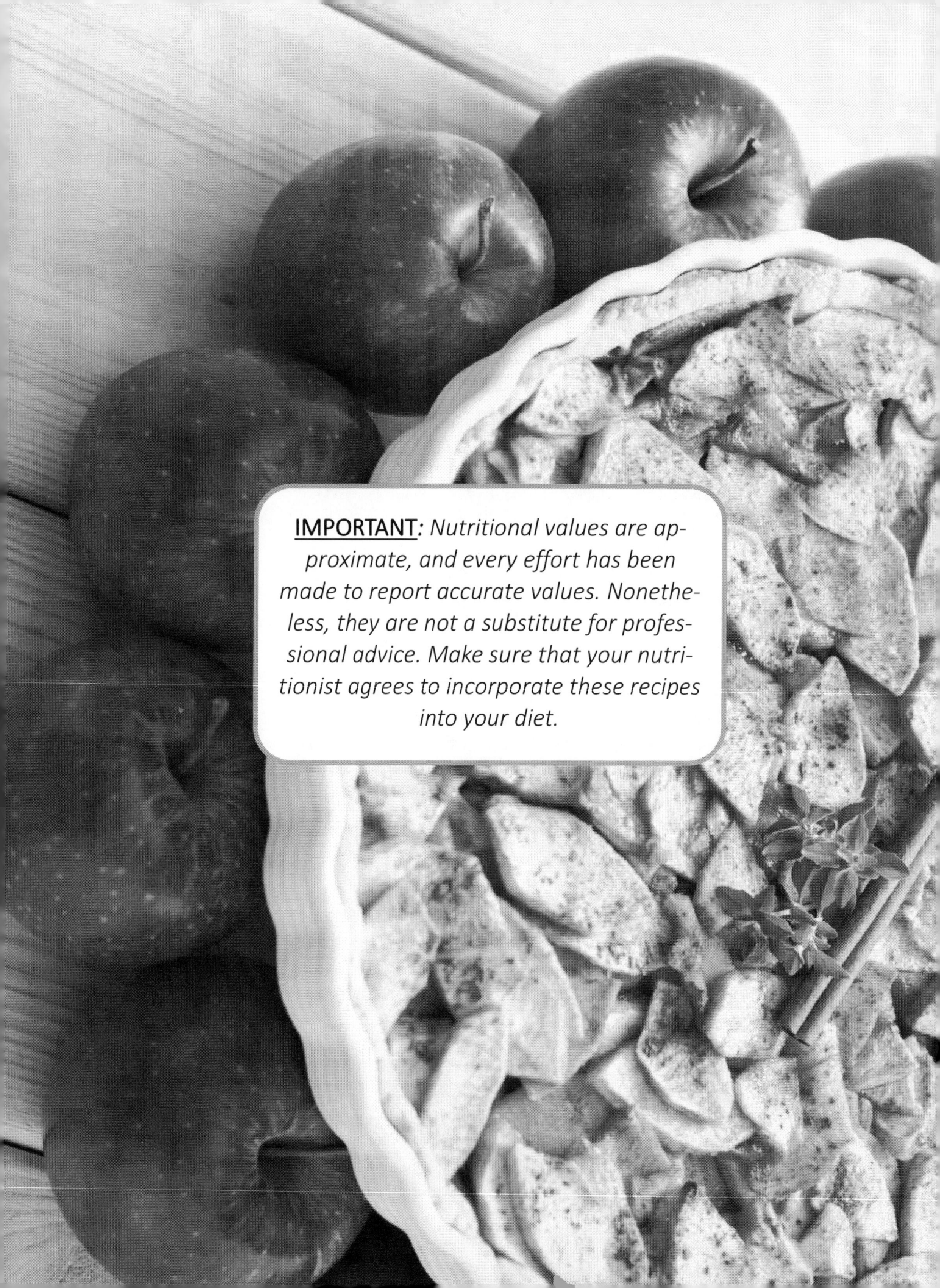

IMPORTANT: *Nutritional values are approximate, and every effort has been made to report accurate values. Nonetheless, they are not a substitute for professional advice. Make sure that your nutritionist agrees to incorporate these recipes into your diet.*

BREAKFAST

The best breakfast is a smile given early in the morning. Throw in one of these recipes and the result is a perfect day.

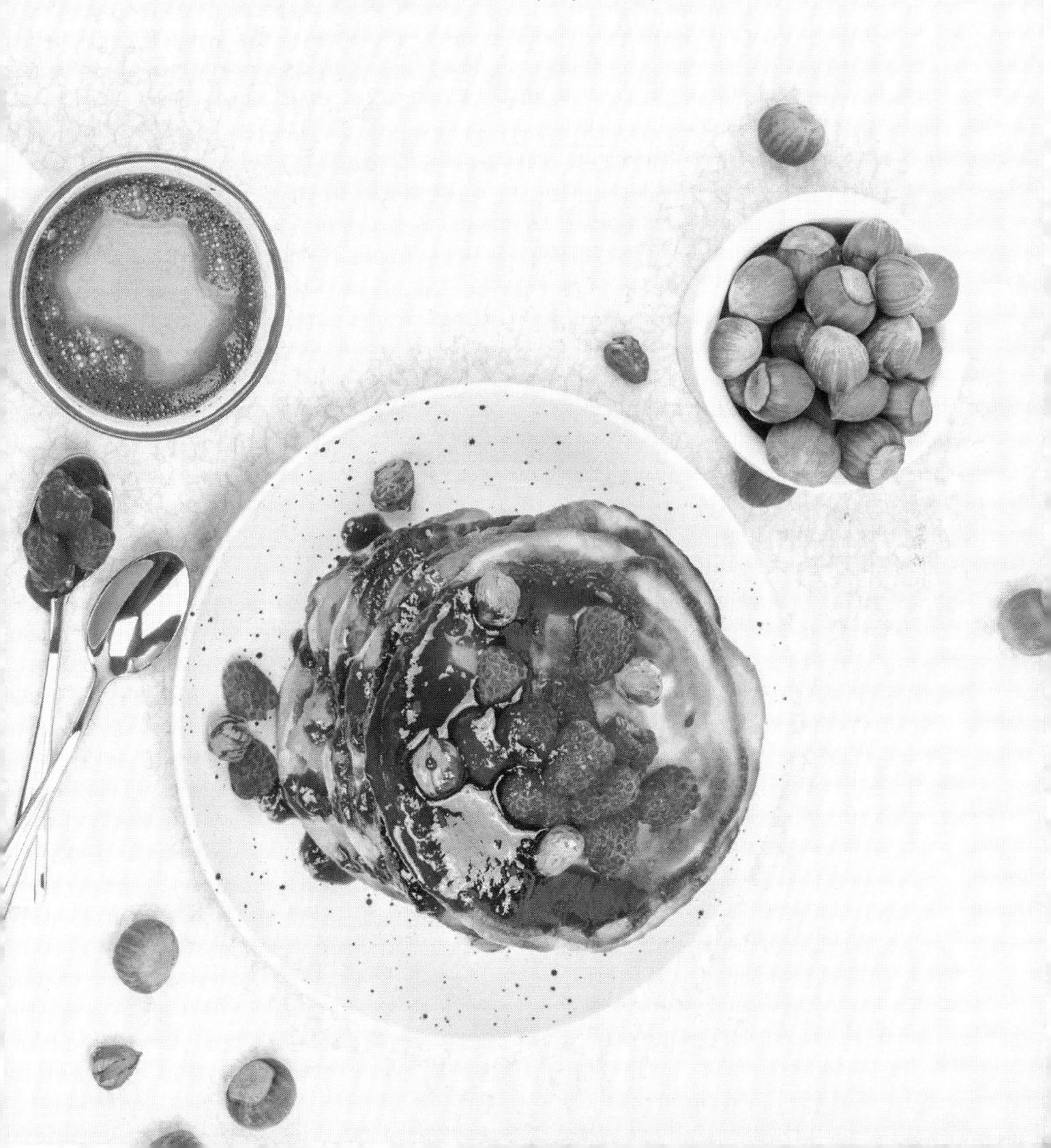

ALMOND AND BLUEBERRY MUFFINS

PREPARATION TIME: 20 MINUTES- **COOKING TIME:** 10 MINUTES- **SERVINGS: 8**

CALORIES: 50, **CARBOHYDRATES:** 20g, **PROTEINS:** 1g, **FAT:** 2g

INGREDIENTS
1 teaspoon apple cider vinegar
1 teaspoon vanilla extract
1 cup almond flour
2 drops of liquid stevia
2 tablespoons butter
3 tablespoons almond milk
1 cup blueberries
Muffin molds
A pinch of salt

DIRECTIONS
1) Put the almond flour in a bowl
2) Add the liquid stevia, salt, and vanilla extract
3) Add the butter, almond milk, and apple cider vinegar
4) Crush the blueberries and add them to the mixture
5) Stir gently with the help of a fork
6) Let the mixture sit for about 5 minutes
7) Heat the air fryer to 350F
8) Prepare the muffin molds
9) Put the mixture into the molds, filling them halfway full
10) Put the muffins in the air fryer and bake them for 10 minutes
11) Let them cool for a few minutes before serving

ALMOND DONUTS

PREPARATION TIME: 5 MINUTES- **COOKING TIME:** 15 MINUTES- **SERVINGS: 8**

CALORIES: 130, **CARBOHYDRATES:** 25g, **PROTEINS:** 2g, **FAT:** 2g

INGREDIENTS
1 teaspoon vanilla extract
1 cup almond flour
2 eggs
3 teaspoons maple syrup
1 tablespoon of baking powder

DIRECTIONS
1) In a bowl, combine all the ingredients
2) Stir until smooth
3) Bake the mixture in the air fryer at 320F for 15 minutes
4) Serve the doughnuts at room temperature

APPLE CAKE

PREPARATION TIME: 15 MINUTES- COOKING TIME: 35 MINUTES- SERVINGS: 8

CALORIES: 130, CARBOHYDRATES: 10g, PROTEINS: 3g, FAT: 8g

INGREDIENTS
- 1 teaspoon butter
- 1 teaspoon cinnamon
- 2 drops of liquid stevia
- 1 roll of puff pastry
- 1 egg
- 2 teaspoons lemon juice
- 2 large apples
- Half teaspoon vanilla extract

DIRECTIONS
1) Sprinkle the baking pan with seed oil
2) Lay out the puff pastry evenly
3) In a bowl, mix vanilla, liquid stevia, cinnamon, lemon juice, and sliced apples
4) On top of the apples, add the chopped butter
5) Cover the apples with more puff pastry
6) Poke holes in the pastry with a knife to let the cooking air escape
7) Brush the top with egg
8) Cover with tin foil
9) Bake in the air fryer at 350F for 25 minutes
10) Remove tin foil and bake for another 10 minutes at 330F.
11) Wait for the cake to cool before tasting it

APPLE TREATS

PREPARATION TIME: 10 MINUTES- COOKING TIME: 25 MINUTES- SERVINGS: 4

CALORIES: 120, CARBOHYDRATES: 12g, PROTEINS: 4g, FAT: 2g

INGREDIENTS
- 2 drops of liquid stevia
- 2 teaspoons coconut oil
- 2 sheets of puff pastry
- 2 small apples

DIRECTIONS
1) Preheat the air fryer to 350F
2) Peel the apples and remove the seeds
3) In a bowl, mix the apples with the liquid stevia
4) Place the mixture on one of the puff pastry sheets
5) Cover it with the second sheet of puff pastry
6) Drizzle the top with coconut oil
7) Bake for 25 minutes at 350F, turning the dough halfway through baking
8) Serve them at room temperature

BANANA AND CHOCOLATE BROWNIES

PREPARATION TIME: 5 MINUTES- **COOKING TIME:** 30 MINUTES- **SERVINGS: 8**

CALORIES: 150, **CARBOHYDRATES:** 20g, **PROTEINS:** 4, **FAT:** 10g

INGREDIENTS
1 ripe banana
1 tablespoon vinegar
1/2 cup cocoa powder
3 large eggs
2 1/2 cups almond flour
1/2 cup coconut oil
Half a teaspoon of baking powder

DIRECTIONS
1) Preheat the air fryer to 350F for 5 minutes
2) Combine all the ingredients
3) Mix until mixture is smooth
4) Bake the mixture for 30 minutes at 350F
5) Serve the brownies freshly cooked for maximum flavor

BANANA BREAD

PREPARATION TIME: 20 MINUTES- **COOKING TIME:** 25 MINUTES- **SERVINGS: 4**

CALORIES: 107, **CARBOHYDRATES:** 10, **PROTEINS:** 6g, **FAT:** 5g

INGREDIENTS
1 teaspoon salt
1 large egg
2 drops of liquid stevia
1 1/2 cups almond flour
3 mashed ripe bananas
1/2 cup melted butter

DIRECTIONS
1) Sprinkle a baking pan with a drop of oil
2) In a large bowl, mix the bananas and liquid stevia
3) In a second bowl, mix the egg, butter, flour, and salt
4) Combine the two compounds
5) Mix well
6) Pour the contents into the baking dish
7) Bake in the air fryer at 300F for 25 minutes
8) Let the banana bread cool for a few minutes and serve it freshly cooked

BANANA CHIPS

PREPARATION TIME: 15 MINUTES- **COOKING TIME:** 15 MINUTES- **SERVINGS: 4**

CALORIES: 35, **CARBOHYDRATES:** 2g, **PROTEINS:** 6g, **FAT:** 3g

INGREDIENTS
- 2 tablespoons of almond flour
- 2 tablespoons cornmeal
- 4 ripe bananas
- 1/2 cup rice flour
- Water as much as needed
- Half a teaspoon of cardamom
- A pinch of salt

DIRECTIONS
1) In a bowl, mix rice flour, cornmeal, almond flour, coconut, cardamom, and salt
2) Add water until the mixture becomes moist and uniform
3) Cut bananas in half, first lengthwise and then widthwise
4) Dip the bananas into the previously prepared mixture
5) Dip them quickly in rice flour
6) Bake them in the air fryer at 350F for 15 minutes
7) Serve them once cooled

BANANA SPLIT

PREPARATION TIME: 15 MINUTES- **COOKING TIME:** 10 MINUTES- **SERVINGS: 4**

CALORIES: 108, **CARBOHYDRATES:** 13g, **PROTEINS:** 5g, **FAT:** 4g

INGREDIENTS
- 1 cup almond flour
- 2 tablespoons chopped hazelnuts
- 2 eggs
- 2 cups breadcrumbs
- 3 tablespoons coconut oil
- 2 drops of liquid stevia
- 4 bananas cut in half
- Optional: vanilla ice cream to taste
- A pinch of cinnamon

DIRECTIONS
1) In a frying pan, heat coconut oil
2) Add the breadcrumbs and air fry for 3-4 minutes
3) Once the bread is golden brown and crispy, let it cool
4) In a bowl, mix the eggs but do not beat them until stiff
5) Sprinkle the bananas with almond flour
6) Dip the bananas in the eggs
7) Add the breadcrumbs
8) Also, add the liquid stevia, hazelnuts, and cinnamon
9) Bake the bananas in the air fryer at 280F for 10 minutes
10) Serve them freshly cooked with some vanilla ice cream

BERRY TACOS

PREPARATION TIME: 5 MINUTES- **COOKING TIME:** 5 MINUTES- **SERVINGS:** 4

CALORIES: 108, **CARBOHYDRATES:** 14, **PROTEINS:** 8g, **FAT:** 4g

INGREDIENTS
2 drops of liquid stevia
2 ready-made tacos
4 tablespoons of berry jam
1/2 cup fresh raspberries
1/2 cup fresh blueberries

DIRECTIONS
1) Sprinkle each taco with two tablespoons of jam
2) Add the blueberries and raspberries
3) Sprinkle the tacos with liquid stevia
4) Bake the tacos at 300F for 5 minutes
5) Serve them freshly cooked

BUTTER COOKIES

PREPARATION TIME: 15 MINUTES- **COOKING TIME:** 10 MINUTES- **SERVINGS:** 4

CALORIES: 70, **CARBOHYDRATES:** 7g, **PROTEINS:** 5g, **FAT:** 2g

INGREDIENTS
2 teaspoons vanilla extract
2 medium eggs
1 3/4 cups hazelnuts
2 drops of liquid stevia
1/2 cup butter
3 cups almond flour
3 tablespoons of baking powder

DIRECTIONS
1) In a small saucepan, heat the butter until it becomes liquid
2) Add the liquid stevia
3) Stir until melted
4) In a bowl, combine the almond flour with the hazelnuts, vanilla extract, baking powder, and eggs
5) Mix well
6) Add the butter and liquid stevia mixture
7) Divide the resulting dough into small servings, so they can fit in the air fryer
8) Bake in the air fryer at 350F for 10 minutes
9) Serve the cookies after they have cooled

CHEESECAKE TREATS

PREPARATION TIME: 60 MINUTES- COOKING TIME: 2 MINUTES- SERVINGS: 4

CALORIES: 60, CARBOHYDRATES: 4g, PROTEINS: 7g, FAT: 6g

INGREDIENTS
1 cup almond flour
2 drops of liquid stevia
3/4 cup cream cheese spread
4 tablespoons of cream
Half a teaspoon of vanilla extract

DIRECTIONS
1) Combine the cream cheese, liquid stevia, cream, and vanilla extract
2) Mix gently for a few minutes
3) Freeze the mixture in the freezer until it solidifies
4) In a bowl, add the almond flour, a pinch of liquid stevia
5) Mix well
6) Thaw the mixture
7) Divide it into 12 cupcakes
8) Dip each treat into the cream
9) Sprinkle each treat with the flour and liquid stevia mixture you just prepared
10) Bake each treat in the air fryer for 2 minutes at a temperature of 300F
11) Serve the treats freshly cooked

CHOCOLATE BALLS

PREPARATION TIME: 15 MINUTES- COOKING TIME: 13 MINUTES- SERVINGS: 4

CALORIES: 65, CARBOHYDRATES: 4, PROTEINS: 14g, FAT: 6g

INGREDIENTS
2 drops of liquid stevia
1/2 cup butter
1/2 cup chocolate cut into 8 pieces
2 tbsp. cocoa powder
3 1/2 cup almond flour
One tablespoon of vanilla extract
A pinch of cinnamon

DIRECTIONS
1) Mix the flour, liquid stevia, cocoa powder, cinnamon, and vanilla extract in a bowl
2) Cut the butter into small pieces and add it to the dough
3) Divide the dough into 8 equal-sized balls
4) Place a piece of chocolate in the center of each sphere
5) Place the spheres in the baking dish and bake them at 350F for 8 minutes
6) Next, lower the temperature to 250F and bake the spheres for another 5 minutes
7) Let them cool completely before serving

CHOCOLATE CAKE

PREPARATION TIME: 10 MINUTES- **COOKING TIME:** 35 MINUTES- **SERVINGS: 4**

CALORIES: 64, **CARBOHYDRATES:** 5g, **PROTEINS:** 9g, **FAT:** 3g

INGREDIENTS
1 teaspoon vanilla extract
1 egg
1 cup flaked coconut
1/2 cup hot water
1/2 cup almond milk
2 drops of liquid stevia
1/2 cup almond flour
1/4 cup olive oil
Half a teaspoon of salt
1 tablespoon of baking powder

DIRECTIONS
1) Preheat the air fryer to 350F
2) In a bowl, mix all the dry ingredients
3) Add the liquids
4) Continue stirring until the mixture is nice and firm
5) Put the mixture in a baking dish and cover it with aluminum foil
6) Make small holes in the surface to allow air to pass through
7) Bake for 35 minutes
8) Remove the aluminum foil and bake for another 10 minutes
9) Serve freshly cooked

CHOCOLATE CHIP COOKIES

PREPARATION TIME: 10 MINUTES- **COOKING TIME:** 12 MINUTES- **SERVINGS: 4**

CALORIES: 40, **PROTEINS:** 1g, **CARBOHYDRATES:** 13g, **FAT:** 3g

INGREDIENTS
1 teaspoon vanilla extract
1 egg
1 cup chocolate pieces
1 1/4 cup almond flour
1/2 cup of butter at room temperature
2 drops of liquid stevia
A pinch of salt

DIRECTIONS
1) Preheat the air fryer by setting the temperature to 350F
2) Melt some butter on the baking sheet you are going to use to bake the cookies
3) In a bowl, mix the liquid stevia, and butter
4) Add the vanilla, and egg and mix vigorously
5) Add the salt and flour
6) Add the chocolate pieces, continuing to mix
7) Move half the dough to the baking pan and carefully spread it evenly
8) With the help of a knife, divide the dough into small cookies
9) Place the baking pan in the air fryer and select the "baking" mode
10) Bake for 12 minutes

CHOCOLATE CREAM

PREPARATION TIME: 5 MINUTES- **COOKING TIME:** 20 MINUTES- **SERVINGS: 4**

CALORIES: 120, **CARBOHYDRATES:** 12g, **PROTEINS:** 18g, **FAT:** 8g

INGREDIENTS	DIRECTIONS
1 teaspoon of chocolate chips 1 cup milk 1/2 cup cream 5 large eggs 2 drops of liquid stevia Whipped cream to taste	1) Mix the milk and cream in a bowl 2) Add the eggs and liquid stevia 3) Bake the mixture at 350F for 20 minutes 4) Divide the mixture into 4 servings and serve the cream freshly cooked

CHOCOLATE CUPS

PREPARATION TIME: 15 MINUTES- **COOKING TIME:** 15 MINUTES- **SERVINGS: 4**

CALORIES: 102, **CARBOHYDRATES:** 3g, **PROTEINS:** 12g, **FAT:** 5g

INGREDIENTS	DIRECTIONS
1 teaspoon vanilla extract 1 cup cocoa powder 2 drops of liquid stevia 0.5oz butter 2 cups coconut cream 2 cups cream cheese	1) Preheat the air fryer to 350F 2) Combine all the ingredients in a bowl 3) Stir until smooth 4) Pour mixture into 3 coffee cups 5) Bake at 350F for 15 minutes 6) Let the cups cool 7) Once they reach room temperature place them in the refrigerator for a few hours 8) Serve them as soon as they are removed from the refrigerator

CHOCOLATE PUDDING

PREPARATION TIME: 10 MINUTES- **COOKING TIME:** 20 MINUTES- **SERVINGS: 4**

CALORIES: 80, **CARBOHYDRATES:** 2g, **PROTEINS:** 7g, **FAT:** 2g

INGREDIENTS	DIRECTIONS
3/4 cup agar agar 1 1/4 cups hot coconut milk 4 tbsp. cocoa powder 2 drops of liquid stevia 1/4 cup water 1 tablespoon vinegar	1) In a bowl, mix milk with liquid stevia and cocoa powder 2) In another bowl, mix the agar agar with water 3) Add the previously prepared mixture 4) Transfer to the air fryer and bake at 350F for 20 minutes 5) Serve the pudding chilled after refrigerating it for a few hours

CINNAMON TOAST

PREPARATION TIME: 10 MINUTES- COOKING TIME: 10 MINUTES- SERVINGS: 4

CALORIES: 60, CARBOHYDRATES: 7g, PROTEINS: 5g, FAT: 2g

INGREDIENTS	DIRECTIONS
12 slices of bread 2 drops of liquid stevia 2 teaspoons cinnamon powder 2 teaspoons vanilla extract 2 cups coconut or seed oil	1) Heat the coconut oil in a small saucepan 2) Mix it with the liquid stevia until smooth 3) Incorporate the other ingredients, except the bread 4) Spread the mixture on the bread 5) Bake the bread at 300F for 5 minutes

COCOA AND ALMOND BARS

PREPARATION TIME: 10 MINUTES- COOKING TIME: 4 MINUTES- SERVINGS: 4

CALORIES: 70, CARBOHYDRATES: 7g, PROTEINS: 19g, FAT: 6g

INGREDIENTS	DIRECTIONS
1 cup peeled almonds 1/2 cup goji berries 1/2 cup cocoa powder 8 pitted dates	1) Combine almonds with cocoa powder and goji berries 2) Mix well 3) Add the dates 4) Blend everything with a food processor 5) Spread the mixture on a sheet of baking paper 6) Bake in the air fryer at 300F for 4 minutes 7) Divide the mixture into smaller servings 8) Wait at least 30 minutes before consuming the bars

COFFEE CAKE

PREPARATION TIME: 10 MINUTES- COOKING TIME: 15 MINUTES- SERVINGS: 4

CALORIES: 97, CARBOHYDRATES: 5g, PROTEINS: 8g, FAT: 3g

INGREDIENTS	DIRECTIONS
1 tablespoon cocoa powder 1 tablespoon coffee powder 1 egg 0.5oz butter 0.5oz almond flour 2 drops of liquid stevia	1) In a bowl, beat the eggs together with the butter and liquid stevia 2) Add the coffee, cocoa powder 3) Stir well 4) Add flour while continuing to mix 5) Bake the batter at 330F for 15 minutes

COOKIE DOUGHNUTS

PREPARATION TIME: 5 MINUTES- **COOKING TIME:** 5 MINUTES- **SERVINGS: 4**

CALORIES: 104, **CARBOHYDRATES:** 3g, **PROTEINS:** 5g, **FAT:** 4g

INGREDIENTS
- 1 teaspoon cinnamon
- 2 cups of your favorite cookies
- 3 tablespoons coconut oil
- 2 drops of liquid stevia

DIRECTIONS
1) Mix the liquid stevia with the cinnamon
2) Make a round hole in the center of the cookies
3) Bake them in the air fryer for 5 minutes at 350F
4) Coat them with coconut oil
5) Dip them in the liquid stevia and cinnamon mixture

CRISPY APPLE CHIPS

PREPARATION TIME: 10 MINUTES- **COOKING TIME:** 8 MINUTES- **SERVINGS: 4**

CALORIES: 15, **CARBOHYDRATES:** 2g, **PROTEINS:** 6g, **FAT:** 0g

INGREDIENTS
- 3 crisp, sweet apples
- 3 to 4 tablespoons of cinnamon
- A pinch of salt

DIRECTIONS
1) Wash the apples well using warm water
2) Choose whether or not to peel the apples according to your taste
3) Heat the air fryer to 400F
4) While you wait for the fryer to reach temperature, cut the apples into rounds
5) In a bowl, mix the salt with the cinnamon
6) Dip the apples in the cinnamon and salt mixture
7) Arrange them in the air fryer without letting them overlap
8) Bake for 8 minutes at 400F, turning them halfway through cooking
9) Once they reach the desired appearance, let them cool
10) Consume them freshly cooked or store them in an airtight container

FRIED BANANAS

PREPARATION TIME: 10 MINUTES- **COOKING TIME:** 10 MINUTES- **SERVINGS:** 4

CALORIES: 102, **CARBOHYDRATES:** 3g, **PROTEINS:** 12g, **FAT:** 5g

INGREDIENTS
2 ripe bananas
2 teaspoons sunflower or avocado oil
Optional: a pinch of salt

DIRECTIONS
1) Heat the air fryer to 400F
2) Cut the bananas into rounds.
3) Mix the oil, salt, and bananas in the basket of the fryer
4) Air fry for 10 minutes, stirring halfway through cooking
5) Serve them freshly cooked
6) They are at their best when drizzled with chocolate cream

FRIED PEACHES

PREPARATION TIME: 130 MINUTES- **COOKING TIME:** 10 MINUTES- **SERVINGS:** 4

CALORIES: 60, **CARBOHYDRATES:** 5g, **PROTEINS:** 12g, **FAT:** 3g

INGREDIENTS
1 tablespoon of olive oil
3/4 cup water
2 tablespoons of brandy
2 egg yolks
1/2 cup almond flour
4 egg whites
4 ripe peaches
A pinch of salt
2 drops of liquid stevia

DIRECTIONS
1) Combine the flour with the egg yolks and salt
2) Mix slowly, adding the water and brandy
3) Let the mixture stand for two hours
4) Boil a pot of water
5) Score an X at the base of each peach
6) Fill another bowl with water and ice
7) Boil each peach for about one minute
8) Place the peaches in cold water, allowing the peel to come off
9) Add the egg whites to the first mixture
10) Dip each peach into the mixture
11) Bake the peaches in the air fryer at 350F for 10 minutes
12) Serve them after sprinkling them with liquid stevia

ORANGE COOKIES

PREPARATION TIME: 20 MINUTES- **COOKING TIME:** 12 MINUTES- **SERVINGS: 4**

CALORIES: 70, **CARBOHYDRATES:** 4g, **PROTEINS:** 5g, **FAT:** 4g

INGREDIENTS

1 teaspoon vanilla extract
1 teaspoon orange zest
1 egg
2 drops of liquid stevia
2 cups butter
1/2 cup almond flour
For the filling:
1 cup cream cheese

DIRECTIONS

1) In a bowl, mix the cream cheese with 1 cup of butter and liquid stevia
2) In another bowl, mix another 1 cup butter with liquid stevia, egg, vanilla extract, and orange zest
3) Add the flour to the second mixture
4) Mix well
5) Pour the mixture into the air fryer
6) Bake at 350F for 12 minutes
7) Let the cookies cool
8) Spread them with the cream from the first bowl
9) Serve them freshly cooked

PEANUT BUTTER AND JELLY DOUGHNUTS

PREPARATION TIME: 75 MINUTES - **COOKING TIME:** 12 MINUTES- **SERVINGS: 4**

CALORIES: 110, **CARBOHYDRATES:** 15g, **PROTEINS:** 19g, **FAT:** 6g

INGREDIENTS

For the doughnuts:
1 teaspoon vanilla extract
1 large egg
1 cup butter
2 drops of liquid stevia
2 tablespoons peanut butter
2 tablespoons milk
2 cups almond flour
2 tablespoons of baking powder
For the frosting:
Salt to taste
A pinch of salt
For the filling:
1 cup strawberry jam or berries

DIRECTIONS

1) Mix all the solid ingredients for the doughnuts in a bowl
2) In another bowl, combine the eggs, melted butter, and vanilla extract
3) Create a hole in the center of the first mixture
4) Combine the mixture with the eggs
5) Use a fork or spatula to mix the ingredients well
6) Place the dough on a piece of baking paper
7) Knead it with your hands until you get a smooth mixture
8) Divide the dough into 4 pieces
9) Give each piece the classic doughnut shape
10) Bake each doughnut in the air fryer at 350F for 12 minutes
11) Fill the doughnuts with jam
12) Combine the ingredients for the glaze in a bowl
13) Drizzle the glaze over the doughnuts
14) Place the doughnuts in the refrigerator
15) Let them rest one hour before serving

PINEAPPLE SWEETS

PREPARATION TIME: 10 MINUTES- **COOKING TIME**: 10 MINUTES- **SERVINGS: 4**

CALORIES: 60, **CARBOHYDRATES**: 7g, **PROTEINS**: 8g, **FAT**: 2g

INGREDIENTS
1 small jar of vanilla yogurt
0.5oz mint leaves
Half a pineapple

DIRECTIONS
1) Peel the pineapple
2) Cut it into pieces of the size you prefer
3) Bake the pineapple at 350F for 10 minutes
4) Meanwhile, mix the yogurt with the mint leaves
5) Serve the pineapple freshly cooked using the yogurt as a sauce

PLUM AND CURRANT CAKE

PREPARATION TIME: 50 MINUTES- **COOKING TIME**: 35 MINUTES- **SERVINGS: 4**

CALORIES: 89, **CARBOHYDRATES**: 6g, **PROTEINS**: 8g, **FAT**: 3g

INGREDIENTS
For the base:
1 cup butter
2 drops of liquid stevia
2 cups rice flour
1/2 cup of almond flour
1/2 cup millet flour
1/4 cup milk
For the filling:
1 tablespoon lemon juice
2 tablespoons cornstarch
2 cups currants
2 drops of liquid stevia
2 1/2 cups of plums
1/2 cup ginger powder

DIRECTIONS
1) In a bowl, mix rice flour with liquid stevia, millet flour, almond flour, rice flour, butter, and milk
2) Set aside a quarter of the dough and place the rest in a container suitable for your air fryer
3) Place the dough in the refrigerator for 30 minutes
4) In another bowl, mix all the ingredients for the filling
5) Pour this mixture over the dough
6) Cover with the remaining quarter of dough
7) Bake at 350F for 35 minutes
8) Let rest and serve the cake at room temperature

POACHED APPLES

PREPARATION TIME: 15 MINUTES- **COOKING TIME**: 10 MINUTES- **SERVINGS**: 4

CALORIES: 80, **CARBOHYDRATES**: 8g, **PROTEINS**: 9g, **FAT**: 2g

INGREDIENTS
- 1 teaspoon grated orange zest
- 1 roll of puff pastry
- Half a large apple, peeled and seedless
- Half a teaspoon of cinnamon
- 2 drops of liquid stevia

DIRECTIONS
1) In a bowl, mix all the ingredients except the puff pastry
2) Cut the puff pastry into 16 squares
3) Put about a teaspoon of mixture in the center of each square
4) Roll each square into a triangle
5) Press on the edges, helping yourself with a little water to seal the dough
6) Set the air fryer to a temperature of 350F
7) Bake the poached apples for 10 minutes
8) Serve them freshly cooked

PUMPKIN COOKIES

PREPARATION TIME: 10 MINUTES- **COOKING TIME**: 15 MINUTES- **SERVINGS**: 4

CALORIES: 30, **CARBOHYDRATES**: 2g, **PROTEINS**: 5g, **FAT**: 2g

INGREDIENTS
- 1 teaspoon vanilla extract
- 1 cup dark chocolate chips
- 1 cup pumpkin pulp
- 1/2 cup water
- 0.5oz butter
- 1/2 cup honey
- 3 cups almond flour
- 3 tablespoons of baking powder

DIRECTIONS
1) In a bowl, mix the flour with the salt and baking powder
2) In a second bowl, mix the pumpkin and the vanilla extract
3) Add the dark chocolate to the second bowl
4) Combine all the preparations in one bowl
5) Bake the cake in the air fryer at 350F for 15 minutes
6) Let it cool and serve at room temperature

SIMPLE COOKIES

PREPARATION TIME: 20 MINUTES- **COOKING TIME:** 12 MINUTES- **SERVINGS: 4**

CALORIES: 40, **CARBOHYDRATES:** 6g, **PROTEINS:** 4g, **FAT:** 7g

INGREDIENTS	DIRECTIONS
1/2 cup butter 1 1/4 cup almond flour 2 drops of liquid stevia	1) Mix the flour with the liquid stevia and butter 2) Cut dough into equal parts giving the shape you like best 3) Put the cookies on the baking sheet 4) Bake at 350F for 12 minutes 5) Let them rest for 10 minutes before serving

SNOW-WHITE CAKE

PREPARATION TIME: 15 MINUTES- **COOKING TIME:** 30 MINUTES- **SERVINGS:** 4

CALORIES: 71, **CARBOHYDRATES:** 4g, **PROTEINS:** 5g, **FAT:** 3g

INGREDIENTS	DIRECTIONS
12 egg whites 2 drops of liquid stevia 1/2 cup melted butter	1) Heat the air fryer to 350F 2) Beat eggs until white and fluffy 3) Add the rest of the ingredients 4) Mix for another minute 5) Put the mixture into a baking dish 6) Bake for 30 minutes at 350F

SWEET POTATO CROQUETTES

PREPARATION TIME: 35 MINUTES- **COOKING TIME:** 14 MINUTES- **SERVINGS: 4**

CALORIES: 40, **CARBOHYDRATES:** 7g, **PROTEINS:** 9g, **FAT:** 1g

INGREDIENTS

1 tablespoon potato starch
1 tablespoon seed oil
5 sweet potatoes
Peanut butter to taste
A pinch of salt
A pinch of garlic powder

DIRECTIONS

1) Bring water to a boil
2) Add potatoes and cook them until they are cooked. Use a fork to check the degree of cooking
3) Transfer the potatoes to a pan and let them cool
4) Grate the potatoes into a bowl
5) Add the potato starch and salt
6) Helping yourself with your hands, create the croquettes. They should come out between 20 and 25 croquettes
7) Sprinkle the basket of the air fryer with a little seed oil
8) Add the croquettes
9) Bake at 350F for about 14 minutes.

VANILLA BLUEBERRY MUFFINS

PREPARATION TIME: 15 MINUTES- **COOKING TIME:** 12 MINUTES- **SERVINGS: 4**

CALORIES: 80, **CARBOHYDRATES:** 6g, **PROTEINS:** 8g, **FAT:** 2g

INGREDIENTS

1 teaspoon vanilla extract
1 cup cream
2 drops of liquid stevia
2 eggs
2 cups fresh blueberries
2 3/4 cups almond flour
1/2 cup sunflower seed oil
Peel and juice of one orange
Muffin molds

DIRECTIONS

1) Combine the oil, cream, eggs, orange juice, and vanilla extract in a bowl
2) In another bowl, combine the flour and liquid stevia
3) Mix them until smooth
4) Combine the two mixtures, mixing them well
5) Preheat the air fryer to 320F
6) Combine the fresh blueberries with the mixture
7) Divide the mixture into the molds
8) Bake the muffins for 12 minutes

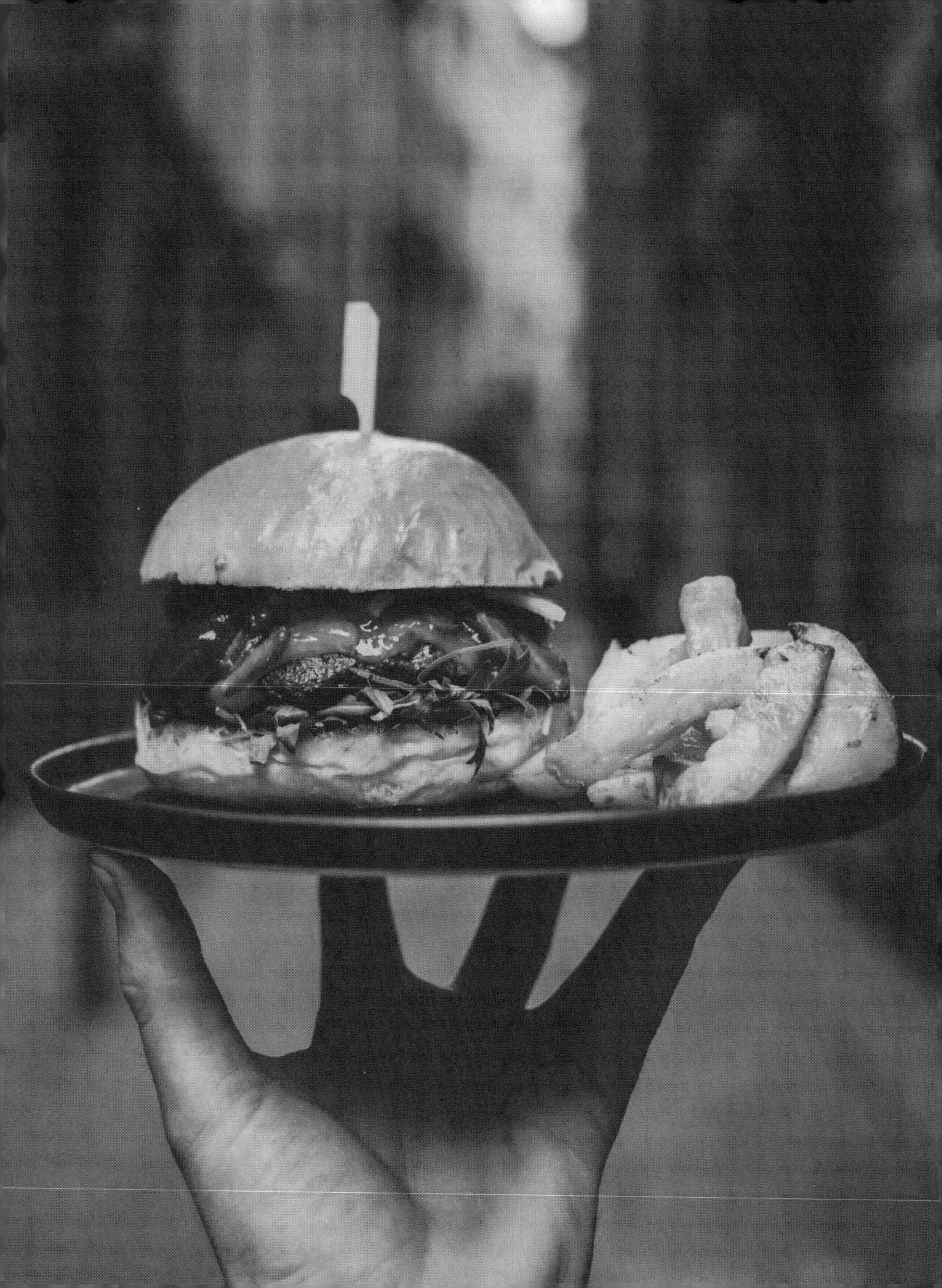

LUNCH

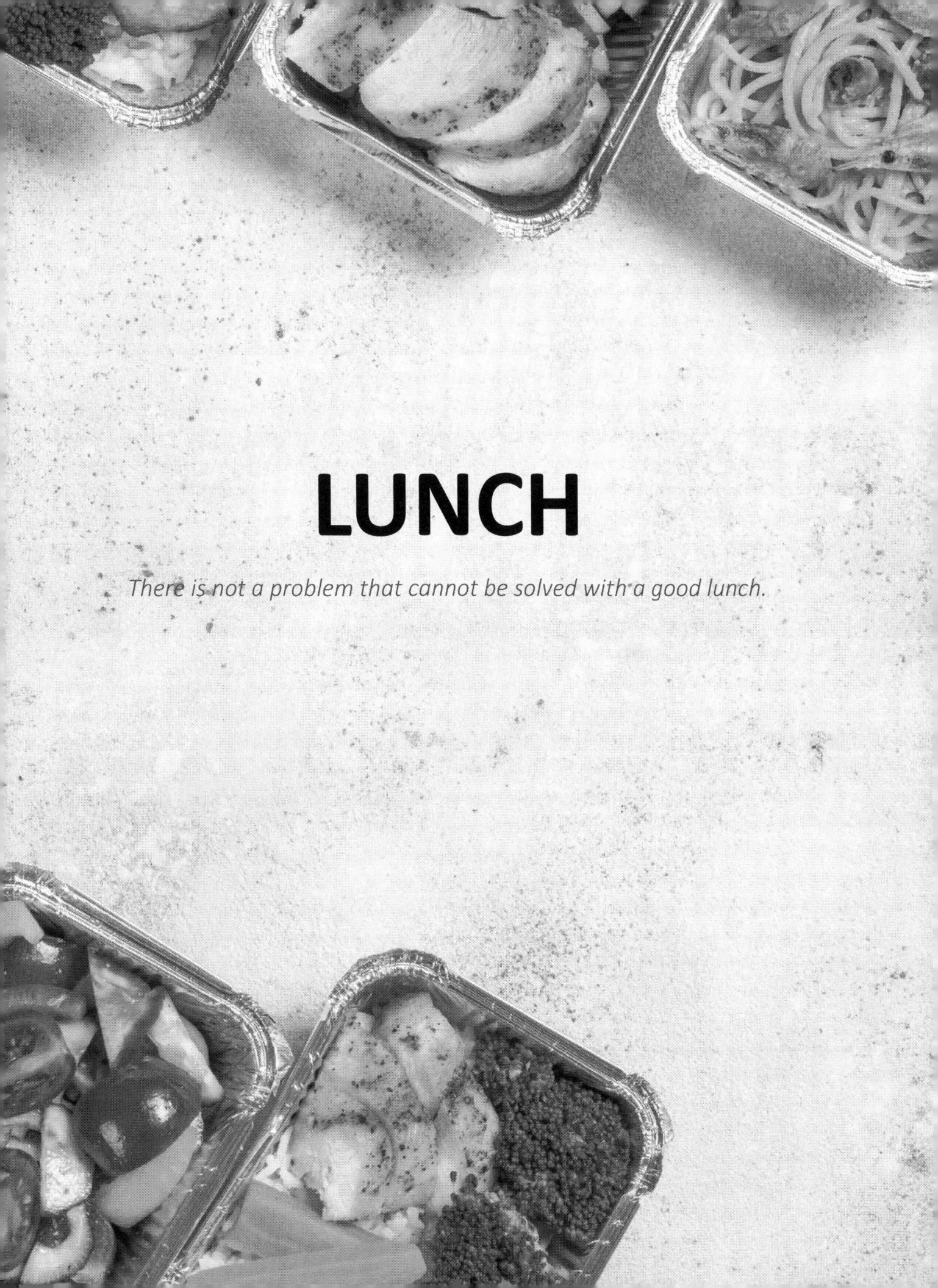

There is not a problem that cannot be solved with a good lunch.

BEEF IN RED WINE REDUCTION

PREPARATION TIME: 25 MINUTES- **COOKING TIME:** 20 MINUTES- **SERVINGS:** 4

CALORIES: 119, **CARBOHYDRATES:** 5g, **PROTEINS:** 13g, **FAT:** 2g

INGREDIENTS
1 tablespoon mustard
1 shallot, finely chopped
0.5oz butter
5 beef steaks from your local butcher's shop
3 cups red wine
Seed oil as much as needed
Salt and pepper to taste

DIRECTIONS
1) Season the beef steaks with salt and pepper
2) Drizzle the beef steaks with oil
3) Cook the steaks in the air fryer at 400F for 10 minutes, turning them halfway through cooking
4) Let the steaks rest for 10 minutes
5) Heat a skillet and cook the shallot together with the butter
6) Pour the wine into the skillet and continue cooking until the wine has completely evaporated
7) Add the mustard, salt, and pepper
8) Continue cooking until the sauce has reduced completely
9) Serve the steaks with the sauce

BEEF TENDERLOIN WITH BUTTER

PREPARATION TIME: 5 MINUTES- **COOKING TIME:** 30 MINUTES- **SERVINGS:** 4

CALORIES: 128, **CARBOHYDRATES:** 4g, **PROTEINS:** 19g, **FAT:** 9g

INGREDIENTS
4 cups of sliced beef tenderloin
1 teaspoon chili powder
1/2 cup butter
Salt to taste

DIRECTIONS
1) Put all the ingredients into the air fryer
2) Mix well
3) Air fry at 400F for 30 minutes
4) Serve freshly cooked

BREADED SOLE

PREPARATION TIME: 15 MINUTES - **COOKING TIME:** 8 MINUTES - **SERVINGS:** 4

CALORIES: 16g, **CARBOHYDRATES:** 3g, **PROTEINS:** 1g, **FAT:** 2g

INGREDIENTS
- 1 onion
- 1 egg
- 2 cups breadcrumbs
- 4 sole fillets
- 1/2 cup grated Parmesan cheese
- A pinch of pepper

DIRECTIONS
1) Preheat the air fryer to 200F
2) In a bowl, chop the onion as finely as possible
3) Add the Parmesan cheese, pepper and egg
4) Dip the sole fillets in the freshly prepared mixture
5) Dip the fillets in the breadcrumbs
6) Bake at 200F for 8 minutes, turning the fillets halfway through cooking
7) Serve the sole freshly cooked

BROCCOLI AND CHEESE CROQUETTES

PREPARATION TIME: 30 MINUTES - **COOKING TIME:** 14 MINUTES - **SERVINGS:** 4

CALORIES: 104, **CARBOHYDRATES:** 1g, **PROTEINS:** 17g, **FAT:** 5g

INGREDIENTS
- 1 egg
- 1 cup parsley
- 0.5oz of minced garlic
- 2 cups of broccoli
- 2 cups breadcrumbs
- 1/2 cup cheese of your choice
- Salt and pepper to taste

DIRECTIONS
1) Using a kitchen blender, grate the broccoli until it looks like rice
2) In a bowl, mix the broccoli with the pepper, salt, egg, cheese, breadcrumbs, and garlic
3) Make 15 croquettes of the same size
4) If necessary, add more breadcrumbs
5) Bake at in the air fryer 380F for 14 minutes, turning the croquettes halfway through cooking
6) Serve them freshly cooked

BROCCOLI AND MUSHROOM OMELET

PREPARATION TIME: 20 MINUTES- **COOKING TIME:** 23 MINUTES- **SERVINGS:** 4

CALORIES: 60, **CARBOHYDRATES:** 5g, **PROTEINS:** 25g, **FAT:** 5g

INGREDIENTS
1 tablespoon olive oil
1 cup porcini mushrooms
1 1/4 cup steamed broccoli
6 eggs
1/2 cup chopped onion
1/2 cup Parmesan cheese
A pinch of pepper
A pinch of salt

DIRECTIONS
1) In the air fryer, using a cooking pan, put all the ingredients except the eggs and Parmesan cheese
2) Air fry at 400F for 8 minutes
3) Meanwhile, in a bowl beat the eggs
4) Mix the eggs with the Parmesan cheese
5) Combine the eggs with the vegetables
6) Air fry everything for another 15 minutes
7) Let the omelet cool 5 minutes before serving

BROCCOLI AND TOFU RISOTTO

PREPARATION TIME: 35 MINUTES- **COOKING TIME:** 15 MINUTES- **SERVINGS:** 4

CALORIES: 100, **CARBOHYDRATES:** 11g, **PROTEINS:** 7g, **FAT:** 4g

INGREDIENTS
1 teaspoon vinegar
1 cup of broccoli
1 cup onions
1 cup frozen peas
2 teaspoons seed oil
2 teaspoons of soy sauce
2 cups carrots
1 1/4 cup rice
Enough water
4 oz tofu

DIRECTIONS
1) Break the tofu into a large bowl
2) Combine all the ingredients except the rice and water
3) Air fry at 250F for 10 minutes, stirring halfway through cooking
4) In a regular pot, cook the rice
5) Combine the two dishes
6) Cook for 5 more minutes, so that the ingredients are well blended
7) Serve freshly cooked

UTTER FRIED CHICKEN

PREPARATION TIME: 330 MINUTES- **COOKING TIME:** 12 MINUTES- **SERVINGS: 4**

CALORIES: 171, **CARBOHYDRATES:** 3g, **PROTEINS:** 9g, **FAT:** 1g

INGREDIENTS
- 1 teaspoon garlic powder
- 1 teaspoon smoked paprika
- 1 cup butter
- 2 cups almond flour
- Half a pound of sliced chicken breast
- Half a teaspoon of onion powder
- Salt and pepper to taste

DIRECTIONS
1) In a bowl, mix the chicken, salt, and pepper
2) Place the chicken in the refrigerator for at least 6 hours, allowing it to season thoroughly
3) In a second bowl, combine the flour, onion, garlic, and smoked paprika
4) Bread the chicken thoroughly in this mixture
5) Bake at 300F for 12 minutes, turning the chicken slices halfway through cooking
6) Serve it freshly cooked

BUTTER SALMON

PREPARATION TIME: 10 MINUTES- **COOKING TIME:** 10 MINUTES- **SERVINGS: 4**

CALORIES: 176, **CARBOHYDRATES:** 2g, **PROTEINS:** 13g, **FAT:** 6g

INGREDIENTS
- 2 salmon fillets
- 2 servings of vegetables of your choice
- 0.5oz melted butter
- Salt and pepper to taste

DIRECTIONS
1) Season each salmon fillet with salt and pepper
2) Sprinkle each salmon fillet with melted butter
3) Bake at 350F for 10 minutes
4) Serve the salmon freshly cooked with steamed vegetables

CAULIFLOWER & CHEESE

PREPARATION TIME: 5 MINUTES- **COOKING TIME:** 6 MINUTES- **SERVINGS: 4**

CALORIES: 57, **CARBOHYDRATES:** 1g, **PROTEINS:** 3g, **FAT:** 4g

INGREDIENTS
- 1 teaspoon of tomato paste
- 1 egg
- 1 cup almond flour
- 1 cup cheese of your choice
- 2 cups cauliflower

DIRECTIONS
1) In a bowl, combine the egg, cheese, cauliflower, tomato paste, and flour
2) Bake the mixture at 400F for 6 minutes
3) Serve it freshly cooked

CHICKEN BREAST

PREPARATION TIME: 5 MINUTES- **COOKING TIME:** 30 MINUTES- **SERVINGS:** 4

CALORIES: 118, **CARBOHYDRATES:** 5g, **PROTEINS:** 25g, **FAT:** 6g

INGREDIENTS
1 cup butter
1 cup cornmeal
2 sliced chicken breasts
2 cups almond flour
4 eggs
A pinch of pepper
A pinch of salt

DIRECTIONS
1) Combine all the ingredients except the chicken in a bowl
2) Preheat the air fryer to 350F
3) Dip each slice of chicken in the mixture
4) Bake at 350F for 30 minutes
5) Serve freshly cooked with steamed vegetables

CHICKEN FAJITA WITH SPICY POTATOES

PREPARATION TIME: 20 MINUTES- **COOKING TIME:** 45 MINUTES- **SERVINGS:** 4

CALORIES: 65, **CARBOHYDRATES:** 5g, **PROTEINS:** 5g, **FAT:** 3g

INGREDIENTS
1 onion
1 teaspoon garlic powder
1 teaspoon oregano
1 teaspoon smoked paprika
1 teaspoon salt
1 yellow bell pepper cut into pieces
1 red bell pepper cut into pieces
3 cups chopped potatoes
2 teaspoons ground chili pepper
3 teaspoons olive oil
3 sliced chicken breasts
4 teaspoons olive oil
8 tortillas

DIRECTIONS
1) In a bowl, combine the spices and oil, mixing well
2) Add the chicken, onion, and peppers
3) Let the chicken marinate in the spices for 10 minutes
4) In another bowl, add the ingredients for the potatoes
5) Air fry the chicken at 400F for 20 minutes, stirring halfway through cooking
6) Air fry potatoes at 350F for 25 minutes, stirring halfway through cooking
7) In a flat pan, cook the tortillas
8) Compose the tortillas
9) Serve them with potatoes

CHICKEN WINGS

PREPARATION TIME: 10 MINUTES- **COOKING TIME:** 20 MINUTES- **SERVINGS: 4**

CALORIES: 60, **CARBOHYDRATES:** 2g, **PROTEINS:** 5g, **FAT:** 8g

INGREDIENTS
- 2 teaspoons paprika
- 2 teaspoons lemon juice
- 1 3/4 cups Greek yogurt
- 1 1/4 cup chicken wings
- Half a teaspoon of chili powder
- A pinch of pepper
- A pinch of salt
- A pinch of garlic

DIRECTIONS
1) In a bowl, add all the ingredients except for the chicken
2) Mix well
3) Dip the chicken in the mixture
4) Place it in the air fryer
5) Air fry the chicken at 280F for 20 minutes, turning it halfway through cooking
6) Serve it freshly cooked

CORDON BLEU

PREPARATION TIME: 25 MINUTES- **COOKING TIME:** 12 MINUTES- **SERVINGS: 4**

CALORIES: 98, **CARBOHYDRATES:** 5g, **PROTEINS:** 21g, **FAT:** 6g

INGREDIENTS
- 1 tablespoon garlic powder
- 1 3/4 cups ham
- 2 cups frozen spinach
- 2 1/2 cups chicken breast
- A pinch of pepper
- A pinch of salt

DIRECTIONS
1) Preheat the air fryer to 350F
2) Dry the chicken by helping yourself with paper towels
3) Cut the chicken into thin slices
4) Add salt and pepper
5) Boil a pot of water and pour in the spinach
6) Once the spinach is cooked, drain it and pat it dry with some kitchen paper
7) Roll the chicken around the ham and spinach, forming rolls
8) Bake at 350F for 12 minutes and serve freshly cooked

CREAMY SALMON

PREPARATION TIME: 5 MINUTES- **COOKING TIME:** 10 MINUTES- **SERVINGS:** 4

CALORIES: 139, **CARBOHYDRATES:** 2g, **PROTEINS:** 16g, **FAT:** 3g

INGREDIENTS
3 tablespoons sour cream
4 salmon fillets
0.5oz Greek yogurt
One tablespoon of olive oil
A pinch of salt

DIRECTIONS
1) Preheat the air fryer to 300F
2) Sprinkle salt over the salmon and add olive oil
3) Air fry for 10 minutes
4) Prepare sauce by mixing yogurt with sour cream and a pinch of salt
5) Serve the salmon freshly cooked with the sauce

FISH AND CHIPS

PREPARATION TIME: 15 MINUTES- **COOKING TIME:** 25 MINUTES- **SERVINGS:** 4

CALORIES: 32, **CARBOHYDRATES:** 7g, **PROTEINS:** 1g, **FAT:** 3g

INGREDIENTS
1 teaspoon of parsley
1 fish fillet of your choice
1 egg
2 cups breadcrumbs
2 1/2 cups potatoes ready to fry
Optional: cocktail sauce to taste
Salt and pepper to taste

DIRECTIONS
1) Preheat the air fryer to 350F
2) Cut the fillet into 4 pieces
3) In a bowl, mix the breadcrumbs with the parsley, egg, pepper, and salt
4) Pass each piece of fillet through the bowl, marinating it thoroughly
5) Air fry the fish at 350F for 15 minutes, turning halfway through cooking
6) Air fry the potatoes at 350F for 10 minutes, turning them every 2 minutes
7) Serve with a drizzle of cocktail sauce

FRIED CHICKEN FILLETS

PREPARATION TIME: 5 MINUTES- **COOKING TIME:** 25 MINUTES- **SERVINGS:** 4

CALORIES: 110, **CARBOHYDRATES:** 2g, **PROTEINS:** 13g, **FAT:** 1g

INGREDIENTS
6 frozen chicken fillets

DIRECTIONS
1) Air fry the chicken fillets in the air fryer at 220F for 25 minutes, turning them halfway through cooking
2) Serve them with a sauce of your choice or vegetables

GARLIC AND SPICE CHICKEN BURGER

PREPARATION TIME: 65 MINUTES- **COOKING TIME:** 7 MINUTES- **SERVINGS:** 4

CALORIES: 114, **CARBOHYDRATES:** 2g, **PROTEINS:** 5g, **FAT:** 8g

INGREDIENTS
- 1 tablespoon garlic powder
- 1 tablespoon mayonnaise
- 1 sliced mozzarella cheese
- 2 eggs
- 0.5oz olive oil
- 1/4 cup water
- 3 chicken burgers

DIRECTIONS
1) Preheat the air fryer to 350F
2) Put all the ingredients except for the mayonnaise in a bowl
3) Mix them well, helping yourself with your hands
4) Cover the bowl and put it in the refrigerator for at least one hour
5) Air fry the burgers for 7 minutes or until golden brown
6) Serve the burgers freshly cooked with a spoonful of mayonnaise

GARLIC PORK TENDERLOINS

PREPARATION TIME: 5 MINUTES- **COOKING TIME:** 25 MINUTES- **SERVINGS:** 4

CALORIES: 61, **CARBOHYDRATES:** 1g, **PROTEINS:** 8g, **FAT:** 3g

INGREDIENTS
- 1 tablespoon garlic powder
- 1 tablespoon coconut oil
- 4 pork tenderloins
- A pinch of pepper
- A pinch of salt

DIRECTIONS
1) Coat the coconut oil, garlic powder, salt, and pepper on the pork tenderloins
2) Bake the fillets in the air fryer at 300F for 25 minutes, turning them halfway through cooking
3) Serve them freshly cooked

HAM AND BELL PEPPER OMELET

PREPARATION TIME: 5 MINUTES- **COOKING TIME:** 15 MINUTES- **SERVINGS:** 4

CALORIES: 101, **CARBOHYDRATES:** 3g, **PROTEINS:** 13g, **FAT:** 4g

INGREDIENTS
- 0.5oz butter
- 0.5oz chopped onion
- 3 eggs
- 1/2 cup diced green peppers
- 1/2 cup ham

DIRECTIONS
1) In the air fryer, put all the ingredients
2) Mix well until mixture is smooth
3) Bake in the air fryer at 300F for 15 minutes
4) Serve freshly cooked

HAMBURGER AND TZATZIKI

PREPARATION TIME: 20 MINUTES- **COOKING TIME:** 20 MINUTES- **SERVINGS:** 4

CALORIES: 120, **CARBOHYDRATES:** 4g, **PROTEINS:** 15g, **FAT:** 5g

INGREDIENTS	DIRECTIONS
For the burgers: 1 teaspoon salt 1 cup chopped onions 2 tablespoons tomato paste 2 cloves of garlic, minced 1/2 cup pitted olives 1 pound of beef A pinch of oregano For the tzatziki: 1 sliced cucumber 2 cups sour cream	1) Preheat the air fryer to 350F 2) In a bowl, place all the ingredients for the burgers 3) Mix well until mixture is smooth 4) Using your hands, shape the burgers 5) Air fry the burgers in the air fryer for 20 minutes, turning them halfway through cooking 6) Prepare the tzatziki by putting all the ingredients in a bowl and mixing well 7) Serve the burgers with a finger of tzatziki as sauce

KEBAB

PREPARATION TIME: 5 MINUTES- **COOKING TIME:** 15 MINUTES- **SERVINGS:** 4

CALORIES: 113, **CARBOHYDRATES:** 2g, **PROTEINS:** 14g, **FAT:** 2g

INGREDIENTS	DIRECTIONS
1 cup onion 2 1/2 cups of minced ground beef One tablespoon of salt A pinch of garlic A pinch of cinnamon A pinch of cardamom	1) Mix all the ingredients until smooth 2) Divide the mixture into 4 equal parts, giving them the shape you like best 3) Bake at 350F for 15 minutes 4) Serve the kebab freshly cooked

LAMB BURGER

PREPARATION TIME: 15 MINUTES- **COOKING TIME:** 14 MINUTES- **SERVINGS:** 4

CALORIES: 123, **CARBOHYDRATES:** 2g, **PROTEINS:** 12g, **FAT:** 4g

INGREDIENTS	DIRECTIONS
2 1/2 cups of lamb meat 1/2 cup onions 1/2 cup of parsley Salt and pepper to taste A pinch of garlic powder A pinch of cinnamon	1) Mix all the ingredients in a bowl 2) Marinate the lamb thoroughly for 10 minutes 3) Divide the meat into 4 equal pieces 4) Bake in the air fryer at 300F for 14 minutes, turning halfway through cooking 5) Serve the burgers freshly cooked

MEATLOAF

PREPARATION TIME: 10 MINUTES- COOKING TIME: 35 MINUTES- SERVINGS: 4

CALORIES: 167, CARBOHYDRATES: 2g, PROTEINS: 14g, FAT: 7g

INGREDIENTS
- 1 tablespoon oil
- 1 egg
- 3/4 cup almond flour
- 3 cups minced pork
- 1/2 heavy whipping cream
- Half a teaspoon of pepper

DIRECTIONS
1) Put all the ingredients in a bowl and mix well, until the mixture is smooth
2) Bake the meatloaf in the air fryer at 300F for 35 minutes
3) Serve it freshly cooked

MINCED MEAT

PREPARATION TIME: 5 MINUTES- COOKING TIME: 12 MINUTES- SERVINGS: 4

CALORIES: 134, CARBOHYDRATES: 3g, PROTEINS: 15g, FAT: 7g

INGREDIENTS
- Half a pound of mince
- One tablespoon of salt
- A pinch of garlic powder
- A pinch of pepper

DIRECTIONS
1) Put the mince in a bowl
2) Add the salt, pepper, and garlic powder
3) Stir well with a wooden spoon.
4) Bake in the air fryer for 12 minutes at 400F, remembering to stir halfway through cooking
5) Use the mixture in your favorite recipes

MOZZARELLA SCHNITZEL

PREPARATION TIME: 40 MINUTES- COOKING TIME: 7 MINUTES- SERVINGS: 4

CALORIES: 67, CARBOHYDRATES: 6g, PROTEINS: 5g, FAT: 2g

INGREDIENTS
- 2 eggs
- 0.5oz extra virgin olive oil
- 1 1/4 cup mince
- 1/4 cup water
- Half a teaspoon of smoked paprika
- BBQ sauce as much as needed
- 4.5oz mozzarella cheese

DIRECTIONS
1) Preheat the air fryer to 350F
2) Using your hands, mix all the ingredients except the olive oil in a bowl
3) Refrigerate for half an hour so the flavors can mix well
4) Give the mixture the typical shape of schnitzels, making at least 4 servings
5) Drizzle each schnitzel with a little olive oil
6) Bake at 350F for 7 minutes
7) Serve the schnitzels freshly cooked

MUSHROOM, BEEF, AND LEEK PIE

PREPARATION TIME: 15 MINUTES- **COOKING TIME**: 7 MINUTES- **SERVINGS**: 4

CALORIES: 179, **CARBOHYDRATES**: 8g, **PROTEINS**: 5g, **FAT**: 3g

INGREDIENTS
1 tablespoon of parsley
1 leek cut into 1 inch rounds
1 roll of puff pastry
1 yolk
2 tablespoons olive oil
2 cups mushrooms
2 cups beef cut into 1 inch pieces
Salt and pepper to taste

DIRECTIONS
1) Preheat the air fryer to 400F
2) Air fry the beef pieces for 5 minutes
3) In a bowl, mix all the ingredients
4) Pass the beef pieces through the mixture, marinating them thoroughly
5) Air fry for an additional 2 minutes at 400F
6) Serve freshly cooked

OREGANO CLAMS

PREPARATION TIME: 10 MINUTES- **COOKING TIME**: 3 MINUTES- **SERVINGS**: 4

CALORIES: 107, **CARBOHYDRATES**: 2g, **PROTEINS**: 7g, **FAT**: 9g

INGREDIENTS
1 teaspoon dried oregano
2 cups breadcrumbs
2 cups salt
25 clams
0.25oz minced garlic
1/2 cup butter
1/2 cup grated Parmesan cheese
1/2 cup parsley

DIRECTIONS
1) Preheat the air fryer to 350F
2) In a bowl, mix breadcrumbs with oregano, basil, Parmesan cheese, and melted butter
3) Add the clams
4) Mix everything
5) Fill the air fryer with salt
6) Lay the clams on top
7) Air fry at 350F for 3 minutes
8) Serve the clams freshly cooked

PAPRIKA AND LEMON GRILLED CHICKEN

PREPARATION TIME: 20 MINUTES- **COOKING TIME:** 42 MINUTES- **SERVINGS:** 4

CALORIES: 131, **CARBOHYDRATES:** 5g, **PROTEINS:** 19g, **FAT:** 3g

INGREDIENTS

- 1/2 cup water
- 2 tablespoons paprika
- 2 lemons
- 4 potatoes
- 5 rosemary leaves
- 2 1/2 cups chicken
- 0.25oz minced garlic
- Salt to taste

DIRECTIONS

1) Combine water with salt, rosemary, and garlic
2) Squeeze the lemons
3) Combine the liquids
4) Salt the chicken and air fry it at 220F for 22 minutes
5) Meanwhile, peel the potatoes and cut them into thick pieces
6) Once the chicken is ready, spread paprika on the surface
7) Air fry at 220F for another 10 minutes.
8) Air fry the potatoes in the air fryer at 350F for 10 minutes
9) Serve the chicken and potatoes freshly cooked

PORCINI MUSHROOM STAKE

PREPARATION TIME: 15 MINUTES- **COOKING TIME:** 18 MINUTES- **SERVINGS:** 4

CALORIES: 60, **CARBOHYDRATES:** 2g, **PROTEINS:** 4g, **FAT:** 3g

INGREDIENTS

- 1 3/4 cups porcini mushrooms
- 0.5oz butter
- 3 beef steaks
- Pepper to taste
- Chopped parsley to taste
- Salt to taste
- A pinch of garlic powder

DIRECTIONS

1) Use a sheet of kitchen paper to dry the steaks and mushrooms
2) Sprinkle both the steak and porcini mushrooms with butter
3) Add garlic powder, salt, and pepper to the steak
4) Air fry both in the air fryer at 400F for 18 minutes, remembering to turn them halfway through cooking
5) Once cooked, scatter the grated parsley and serve

PORK RIBS

PREPARATION TIME: 10 MINUTES- **COOKING TIME:** 14 MINUTES- **SERVINGS:** 4

CALORIES: 84, CARBOHYDRATES: 1g, PROTEINS: 8g, FAT: 2g

INGREDIENTS	DIRECTIONS
1 teaspoon garlic powder 1 teaspoon paprika 1 tablespoon olive oil 2 pork ribs A pinch of pepper A pinch of salt	1) Coat the ribs with olive oil 2) Add the salt, paprika, pepper, and garlic 3) Bake in the air fryer at 350F for 14 minutes, turning halfway through cooking 4) Serve the ribs freshly cooked

ROAST BEEF

PREPARATION TIME: 5 MINUTES- **COOKING TIME:** 45 MINUTES- **SERVINGS:** 4

CALORIES: 165, CARBOHYDRATES: 5g, PROTEINS: 17g, FAT: 3g

INGREDIENTS	DIRECTIONS
1.5lbs roast beef 2 tablespoons of mayonnaise	1) Sprinkle the roast beef with mayonnaise 2) Air fry in the air fryer at 350F for 45 minutes 3) Cut the roast beef into slices 4) Serve freshly cooked

SAUSAGE AND VEGETABLE SANDWICH

PREPARATION TIME: 10 MINUTES- **COOKING TIME:** 25 MINUTES- **SERVINGS:** 4

CALORIES: 126, CARBOHYDRATES: 1g, PROTEINS: 13g, FAT: 2g

INGREDIENTS	DIRECTIONS
1 chopped onion 2 tablespoons of seed oil 2 sliced tomatoes 4 hamburger buns 4 diced bell peppers 4 sausages Mayonnaise to taste	1) Air fry the peppers at 250F for 5 minutes 2) Air fry onions and tomatoes at 250F for 5 minutes 3) Air fry the sausages at 250F for 15 minutes 4) Prepare the sandwiches by dividing the ingredients equally 5) Serve them with mayonnaise

SEASONED COD FILLETS

PREPARATION TIME: 10 MINUTES- **COOKING TIME:** 20 MINUTES- **SERVINGS:** 4

CALORIES: 60, **CARBOHYDRATES:** 4g, **PROTEINS:** 15g, **FAT:** 3g

INGREDIENTS	DIRECTIONS
2 cod fillets Salt and pepper to taste A pinch of garlic powder A pinch of turmeric powder A pinch of ginger powder	1) Dry the codfish with kitchen paper 2) In a bowl, mix the powders 3) Dip the cod in the mixture, letting it marinate for a few minutes 4) Air fry at 350F for 15 minutes 5) Increase the temperature to 400F and air fry for another 5 minutes 6) Serve the cod freshly cooked

SPICY HAMBURGER

PREPARATION TIME: 10 MINUTES- **COOKING TIME:** 10 MINUTES- **SERVINGS:** 4

CALORIES: 95, **CARBOHYDRATES:** 1g, **PROTEINS:** 14g, **FAT:** 3g

INGREDIENTS	DIRECTIONS
1 egg 1 cup almond flour 2 1/2 cups ground pork Salt and pepper to taste	1) Add all the ingredients into a bowl 2) Mix until a homogeneous mixture is created 3) Make two or more burgers of equal size 4) Cook the burgers in the air fryer at 350F for 10 minutes, turning them halfway through cooking 5) Serve the burgers with some steamed vegetables or potatoes

TASTY SALMON

PREPARATION TIME: 10 MINUTES- **COOKING TIME:** 11 MINUTES- **SERVINGS:** 4

CALORIES: 98, **CARBOHYDRATES:** 3g, **PROTEINS:** 13g, **FAT:** 5g

INGREDIENTS	DIRECTIONS
1 teaspoon garlic powder 1 teaspoon onion powder 1 teaspoon paprika 1 teaspoon pepper 2 tablespoons olive oil 2 salmon fillets Salt and pepper to taste	1) Mix the spices in a bowl 2) Drizzle the salmon fillets with the oil 3) Dip the salmon fillets in the spices 4) Air fry them at 300F for 11 minutes, flipping them halfway 5) Serve them freshly cooked

TOFU WITH VEGETABLES

PREPARATION TIME: 5 MINUTES- **COOKING TIME:** 14 MINUTES- **SERVINGS:** 4

CALORIES: 174, CARBOHYDRATES: 12g, PROTEINS: 3g, FAT: 4g

INGREDIENTS
- 1 tomato cut into pieces
- 2 steamed broccoli
- 2 cups sliced tofu
- 3 carrots cut into pieces and steamed
- Salt and pepper to taste
- A pinch of parsley
- A pinch of thyme

DIRECTIONS
1) In the air fryer, put all the ingredients except the tofu
2) Mix well
3) Cook at 350F for 10 minutes, stirring often
4) Add the tofu and cook for another 4 minutes
5) Serve freshly cooked

TURKEY AND AVOCADO BURGER

PREPARATION TIME: 10 MINUTES- **COOKING TIME:** 15 MINUTES- **SERVINGS:** 4

CALORIES: 112, CARBOHYDRATES: 4g, PROTEINS: 18g, FAT: 3g

INGREDIENTS
- 1 avocado peeled, pitted, and cut into pieces
- 2 tablespoons of mayonnaise
- 2 1/2 cups turkey meat
- 1/2 cup green peppers
- A pinch of pepper
- A pinch of salt

DIRECTIONS
1) In a bowl, mix the meat with salt, green pepper, pepper, and mayonnaise
2) Scoop out 4 burgers
3) Air fry the burgers at 350F for 15 minutes
4) Serve the burgers freshly cooked with a slice of avocado on top

TURKEY WINGS

PREPARATION TIME: 5 MINUTES- **COOKING TIME:** 25 MINUTES- **SERVINGS:** 4

CALORIES: 60, CARBOHYDRATES: 3g, PROTEINS: 12g, FAT: 15g

INGREDIENTS
- 2 1/2 cups turkey wings
- Half a tablespoon of olive oil
- Salt and pepper to taste

DIRECTIONS
1) Preheat the air fryer to 350F
2) Sprinkle turkey wings with salt, pepper, and olive oil
3) Air fry for 25 minutes at 350F, flipping the turkey halfway through cooking
4) Serve the wings freshly cooked

VEGETARIAN TOAST

PREPARATION TIME: 5 MINUTES- **COOKING TIME**: 15 MINUTES- **SERVINGS**: 4

CALORIES: 132, **CARBOHYDRATES**: 2g, **PROTEINS**: 13g, **FAT**: 2g

INGREDIENTS
1 onion
1 tablespoon olive oil
1 red bell pepper
1 green bell pepper
1 cup cream cheese
0.5oz butter
2 cups mushrooms
3 slices of bread

DIRECTIONS
1) Mix the mushrooms and peppers in a bowl
2) Add the oil and chopped onion
3) Continue stirring until the mixture is smooth
4) Bake the mixture in the air fryer at 350F for 10 minutes
5) Spread the butter on the bread slices
6) Bake the bread slices at 350F for 5 minutes
7) Assemble the toast and serve freshly cooked

WHITE WINE CHICKEN BREAST

PREPARATION TIME: 30 MINUTES- **COOKING TIME**: 30 MINUTES- **SERVINGS**: 4

CALORIES: 171, **CARBOHYDRATES**: 3g, **PROTEINS**: 12g, **FAT**: 3g

INGREDIENTS
1/2 cup white wine
4 chicken breasts
1/2 cup seed oil
1/2 cup coconut milk
Half a teaspoon of salt
A pinch of garlic
A pinch of pepper
A pinch of grated ginger
A handful of thyme leaves

DIRECTIONS
1) Heat the oil in a pan and add the garlic
2) Cook until the garlic turns golden
3) Remove the pot from the heat
4) Add the coconut oil and white wine
5) Add the thyme, salt, ginger, and pepper
6) Put the mixture in a bowl
7) Dip the chicken breasts in the sauce
8) Air fry the chicken breasts at 250F for 30 minutes
9) Consume them freshly cooked

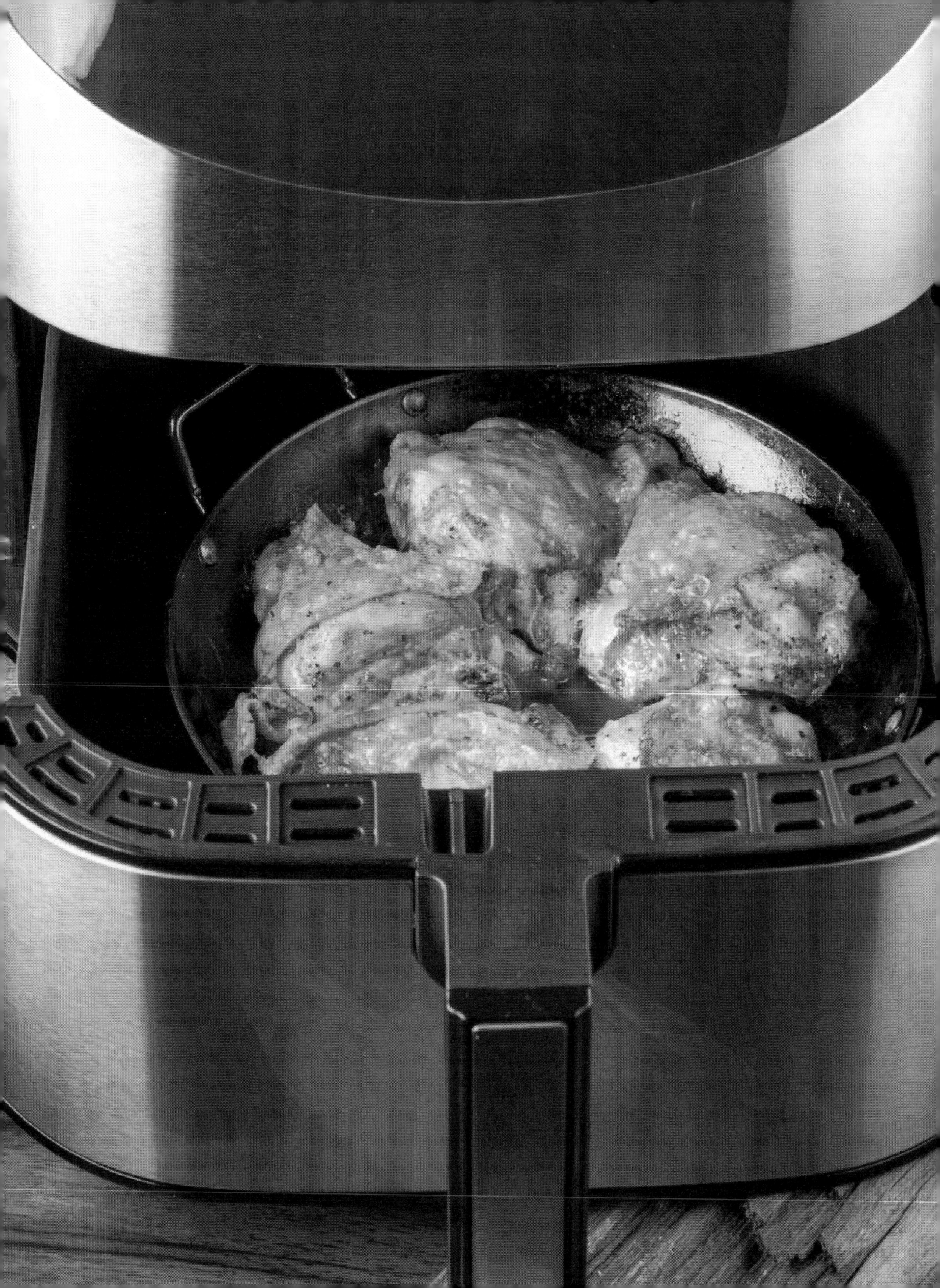

DINNER

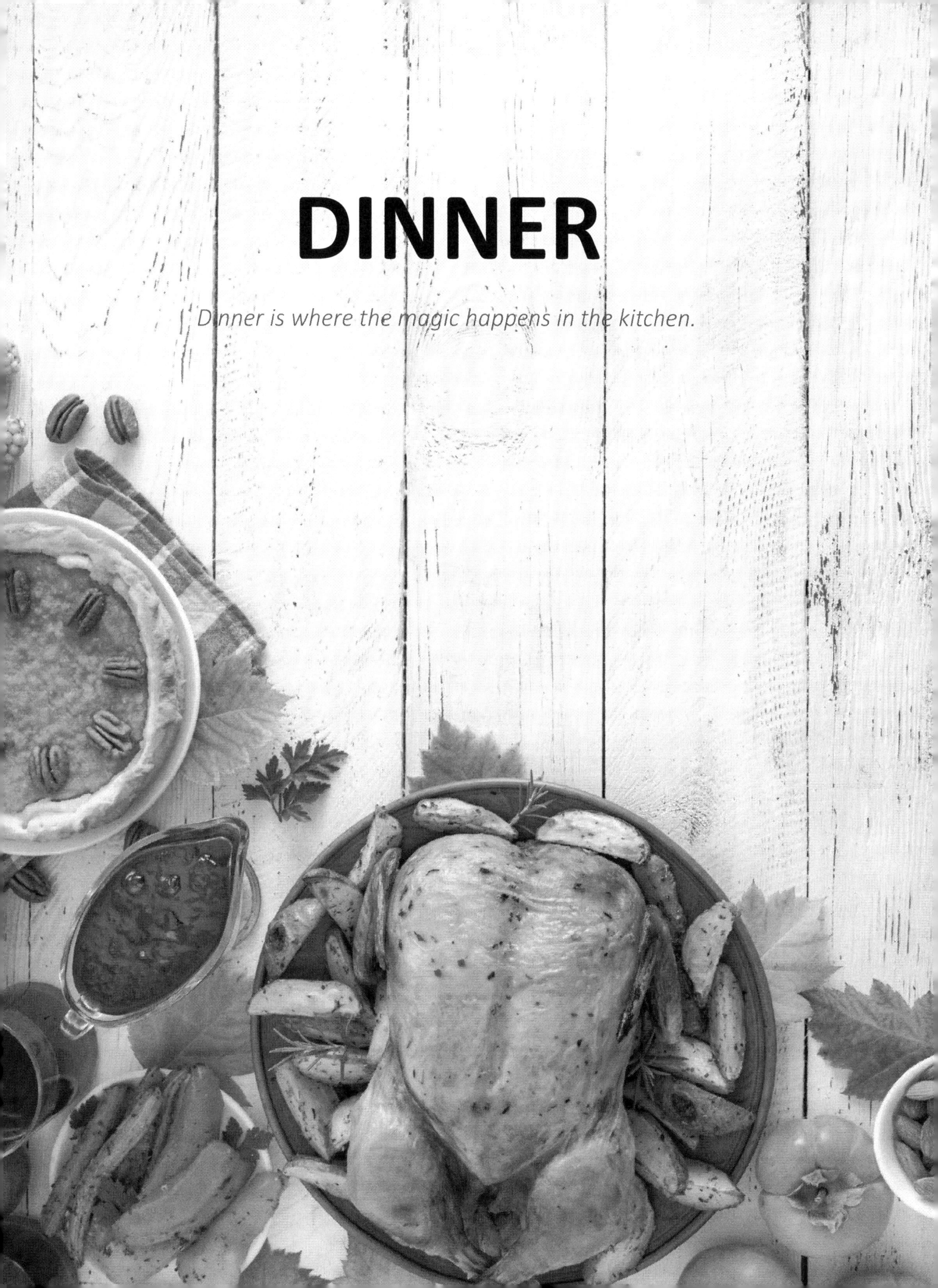

Dinner is where the magic happens in the kitchen.

"CHIPOTLE" STEAKS

PREPARATION TIME: 35 MINUTES- **COOKING TIME:** 10 MINUTES- **SERVINGS:** 4

CALORIES: 167, **CARBOHYDRATES:** 7g, **PROTEINS:** 13g, **FAT:** 2g

INGREDIENTS
3 cups of sliced beef
A pinch of garlic powder
A pinch of cocoa powder
A pinch of coffee
A pinch of onion powder
A pinch of paprika
A pinch of chili pepper
A pinch of salt

DIRECTIONS
1) In a bowl, mix all the powders
2) Dip the steaks in the powder mix you just prepared
3) Let the steaks rest for 30 minutes
4) Air fry the steaks at 400F for 10 minutes, turning them halfway through cooking
5) Serve them freshly cooked

BEEF AND BEANS

PREPARATION TIME: 5 MINUTES- **COOKING TIME:** 8 MINUTES- **SERVINGS:** 4

CALORIES: 78, **CARBOHYDRATES:** 0g, **PROTEINS:** 9g, **FAT:** 4g

INGREDIENTS
1 onion
0.5oz fresh parsley
1 cup drained borlotti beans
3 tomatoes cut into pieces
4 beef steaks
Salt and pepper to taste

DIRECTIONS
1) Preheat the air fryer to 350F
2) Air fry the steaks for 3 minutes
3) Add the other ingredients
4) Air fry for another 5 minutes
5) After cooking, add a pinch of salt and pepper
6) Serve the steaks freshly cooked

BEEF KEBAB

PREPARATION TIME: 40 MINUTES- **COOKING TIME:** 10 MINUTES- **SERVINGS:** 4

CALORIES: 154, **CARBOHYDRATES:** 2g, **PROTEINS:** 15g, **FAT:** 4g

INGREDIENTS
1 onion
1 tablespoon ketchup
1 tablespoon of mayonnaise
1 tablespoon hot sauce
3 cups of beef
2 tomatoes
4 salad leaves
Salt and pepper to taste

DIRECTIONS
1) In a bowl, add the meat, salt, pepper, and chopped onion
2) Mix the ingredients well
3) Let them rest in the refrigerator for 30 minutes
4) Divide the mixture into 4 servings
5) Cook each portion in the air fryer at 350F for 10 minutes and serve with salad and tomatoes

BEEF TACOS

PREPARATION TIME: 25 MINUTES- **COOKING TIME:** 12 MINUTES- **SERVINGS: 4**

CALORIES: 148, **CARBOHYDRATES:** 1g, **PROTEINS:** 4g, **FAT:** 1g

INGREDIENTS
- 1 tablespoon olive oil
- 16 ready-made tacos
- 3 cups minced ground beef
- 2 cloves of garlic
- Half a finely chopped onion
- A pinch of pepper
- A pinch of salt

DIRECTIONS
1) Preheat the air fryer to 400F
2) Add the garlic and onions to a small pan
3) Cook them until crispy
4) Add the salt, pepper, and beef
5) Cook until the mince has broken up nicely
6) Keep stirring for a few minutes
7) Air fry at 400F for 8 minutes
8) Stir and air fry for another 4 minutes
9) In a skillet, heat the tacos until crispy
10) Season the tacos with the mixture
11) Serve them freshly cooked

CALAMARI SKEWERS IN VERMOUTH

PREPARATION TIME: 70 MINUTES- **COOKING TIME:** 5 MINUTES- **SERVINGS:** 4

CALORIES: 129, **CARBOHYDRATES:** 5g, **PROTEINS:** 6g, **FAT:** 2g

INGREDIENTS
- 1 lemon cut into wedges
- 2 cloves of garlic
- 5 tablespoons olive oil
- 1/4 cup vermouth
- 1/2 cup calamari
- Salt and pepper to taste

DIRECTIONS
1) Preheat the air fryer to 400F
2) In a bowl, mix the calamari with the vermouth, olive oil, garlic, salt, and pepper
3) Place the calamari in the refrigerator and let them marinate for an hour
4) Remove the calamari from the refrigerator.
5) Drain the marinade
6) Poke a small hole in the center of each calamari with the help of a toothpick
7) Air fry the squid for 5 minutes, turning them halfway through cooking
8) Insert the squid into the skewers
9) Serve them with a lemon wedge

CAULIFLOWER BALLS

PREPARATION TIME: 15 MINUTES- **COOKING TIME:** 5 MINUTES- **SERVINGS: 4**

CALORIES: 104, CARBOHYDRATES: 3g, PROTEINS: 5g, FAT: 3g

INGREDIENTS
1 tablespoon coconut flour
1 tablespoon of seed oil
1 mozzarella cheese
1 yolk
2 cups cauliflower
1/2 cup cream cheese
A pinch of pepper
A pinch of salt

DIRECTIONS
1) In a bowl, mix the cauliflower with the mozzarella, egg yolk, coconut flour, salt, pepper, and cream cheese
2) Keep stirring until you get a smooth mixture
3) Create small spheres with the dough you just made
4) Bake the cauliflower balls in the air fryer at 400F for 5 minutes.
5) Serve them freshly cooked or at room temperature

CHEESE PORK CHOPS

PREPARATION TIME: 10 MINUTES- **COOKING TIME:** 20 MINUTES- **SERVINGS: 4**

CALORIES: 142, CARBOHYDRATES: 1g, PROTEINS: 5g, FAT: 2g

INGREDIENTS
1 1/2 cup Parmesan cheese
0.5oz butter
0.5oz seed oil
8 pork steaks
A pinch of pepper
A pinch of salt

DIRECTIONS
1) In a bowl, mix the butter, spices, Parmesan cheese, and oil
2) Dip the steaks in the mixture
3) Air fry them at 350F for 20 minutes
4) Serve the steaks freshly cooked

CHICKEN SLICES WITH PEPPERS

PREPARATION TIME: 5 MINUTES- **COOKING TIME:** 15 MINUTES- **SERVINGS: 4**

CALORIES: 141, CARBOHYDRATES: 4g, PROTEINS: 8g, FAT: 3g

INGREDIENTS
2 bell peppers of the color you prefer
4 slices of chicken
1/2 cup butter
A pinch of pepper
A pinch of salt

DIRECTIONS
1) In the air fryer put the chicken slices with the butter, garlic, peppers, salt, and pepper
2) Air fry everything at 250F for 15 minutes, stirring it halfway through

CLASSIC SCHNITZEL

PREPARATION TIME: 10 MINUTES- **COOKING TIME:** 20 MINUTES- **SERVINGS:** 4

CALORIES: 157, **CARBOHYDRATES:** 3g, **PROTEINS:** 28g, **FAT:** 2g

INGREDIENTS
1 tablespoon garlic powder
1 tablespoon onion powder
2 eggs
2 cups almond flour
4 pork steaks
1/2 cup Parmesan cheese
A pinch of pepper
A pinch of salt

DIRECTIONS
1) Preheat the air fryer to 350F
2) In a bowl, mix the Parmesan cheese, onion powder, garlic powder, salt, and pepper
3) Add eggs and mix further
4) Dip the steaks into the mixture
5) Dip the steaks in the flour
6) Cook the steaks at 350F for 20 minutes
7) Serve them freshly cooked

COCONUT-FLAVORED BRUSSELS SPROUTS

PREPARATION TIME: 15 MINUTES- **COOKING TIME:** 2 MINUTES- **SERVINGS:** 4

CALORIES: 140, **CARBOHYDRATES:** 5g, **PROTEINS:** 6g, **FAT:** 3g

INGREDIENTS
1 tablespoon coconut oil
1 celery
2 cups coconut cream
1 1/4 cup Brussels sprouts
Salt and pepper to taste

DIRECTIONS
1) Cook the celery and Brussels sprouts in a pot full of water
2) Drain them in a bowl
3) Add the other ingredients
4) Air fry them at 250F for 2 minutes
5) Consume them freshly cooked

COD FILLETS WITH PARMESAN CHEESE

PREPARATION TIME: 15 MINUTES- **COOKING TIME:** 10 MINUTES- **SERVINGS:** 4

CALORIES: 103, **CARBOHYDRATES:** 5g, **PROTEINS:** 1g, **FAT:** 4g

INGREDIENTS
1 teaspoon garlic powder
1 egg
2 cups Parmesan cheese
4 cod fillets
A pinch of pepper
A pinch of salt

DIRECTIONS
1) Preheat the air fryer to 350F
2) In a bowl, mix Parmesan cheese with egg and garlic powder
3) On the cooking rack, spice the cod fillets with salt and pepper
4) Dip the fillets in the egg and Parmesan mixture
5) Bake the fillets at 350F for 10 minutes, turning them halfway through cooking
6) Let the fillets cool for 5 minutes

FISH TACOS

PREPARATION TIME: 20 MINUTES- **COOKING TIME**: 5 MINUTES- **SERVINGS**: 4

CALORIES: 129, **CARBOHYDRATES**: 5g, **PROTEINS**: 7g, **FAT**: 1g

INGREDIENTS
- 1 tablespoon apple cider vinegar
- 1 tablespoon olive oil
- 1 tablespoon chili pepper
- 1 tablespoon lime juice
- 1.5lbs trout fillets
- 2 1/2 cups cabbage
- 1/2 cup almond flour
- 8 ready-made tacos
- A pinch of pepper
- A pinch of salt

DIRECTIONS
1) Preheat the air fryer to 350F
2) Mix the cabbage, chili, lime juice, olive oil, vinegar, salt, and pepper in a bowl
3) In another bowl, put the flour
4) Dip the trout pieces in the flour
5) Air fry the fish for 5 minutes
6) Mix the fish pieces with the previously prepared cap
7) Heat the tacos in a skillet
8) Season the tacos with the rest of the ingredients
9) Serve them freshly cooked

FLOUNDER FILLETS WITH PARMESAN CHEESE

PREPARATION TIME: 10 MINUTES- **COOKING TIME**: 11 MINUTES- **SERVINGS**: 4

CALORIES: 135, **CARBOHYDRATES**: 4g, **PROTEINS**: 13g, **FAT**: 4g

INGREDIENTS
- 1 egg
- 1 cup Parmesan cheese
- 2 flounder fillets
- A pinch of pepper
- A pinch of fresh parsley
- A pinch of salt

DIRECTIONS
1) Preheat the air fryer to 350F
2) Mix the Parmesan cheese and parsley
3) Add the egg, pepper, and salt
4) Pass the flounder fillets through the mixture until they are well seasoned on both sides
5) Air fry the fillets for 11 minutes or until the skin is opaque
6) Serve the fillets freshly cooked

FRIED SARDINES

PREPARATION TIME: 10 MINUTES- **COOKING TIME:** 12 MINUTES- **SERVINGS:** 4

CALORIES: 138, **CARBOHYDRATES:** 3g, **PROTEINS:** 12g, **FAT:** 3g

INGREDIENTS
- 1 teaspoon vinegar
- 1 tablespoon oil
- 1 tablespoon lemon juice
- 1/2 cup sardines
- Salt and pepper to taste

DIRECTIONS
1) Heat the air fryer to 350F
2) In a bowl, sprinkle sardines with oil, vinegar, lemon juice, salt, and pepper
3) Place the marinated sardines in the air fryer
4) Air fry the sardines for 12 minutes, turning them halfway through cooking
5) Serve them while still hot

GARLIC CALAMARI

PREPARATION TIME: 35 MINUTES- **COOKING TIME:** 4 MINUTES- **SERVINGS:** 4

CALORIES: 162, **CARBOHYDRATES:** 1g, **PROTEINS:** 3g, **FAT:** 2g

INGREDIENTS
- 0.5oz fresh basil
- 0.5oz grated ginger
- 0.25oz minced garlic
- 1/2 cup calamari

DIRECTIONS
1) Preheat the air fryer to 400F
2) Mix all the ingredients in a bowl
3) Let the calamari rest for 30 minutes
4) Air fry the calamari for 4 minutes or until they turn white
5) Serve them hot

GERMAN-STYLE SCHNITZEL

PREPARATION TIME: 20 MINUTES- **COOKING TIME:** 22 MINUTES- **SERVINGS:** 4

CALORIES: 179, **CARBOHYDRATES:** 3g, **PROTEINS:** 5g, **FAT:** 3g

INGREDIENTS
- 1 egg
- 1 cup almond flour
- 1 cup breadcrumbs
- 3 pretzels
- 3 cups chicken breast
- A pinch of pepper
- A pinch of chili pepper
- A pinch of salt

DIRECTIONS
1) Use a meat tenderizer to make the chicken slices extremely thin
2) In a bowl, beat the egg
3) In another bowl, place the flour
4) In a third bowl, mix the breadcrumbs with the salt, pepper, and chili pepper
5) Dip the chicken slices in the flour
6) Dip the chicken in the egg
7) Dip the chicken in the breadcrumbs
8) Air fry at 280F for 22 minutes, turning the schnitzel halfway through cooking

GNOCCHI WITH PARMESAN CHEESE AND CAULIFLOWER

PREPARATION TIME: 25 MINUTES- **COOKING TIME:** 4 MINUTES- **SERVINGS:** 4

CALORIES: 104 **CARBOHYDRATES:** 7g, **PROTEINS:** 7g, **FAT:** 8g

INGREDIENTS
1 yolk
1 3/4 cups Parmesan cheese
0.5oz butter
1/2 cup cauliflower
1/2 cup almond flour
One tablespoon of cream cheese
A pinch of pepper

DIRECTIONS
1) Boil the cauliflower
2) Using a food processor, chop it until it is uniform and very small pieces
3) Place the cauliflower on a kitchen towel
4) Squeeze it to squeeze out excess water
5) Transfer the cauliflower to a bowl
6) Add the Parmesan cheese, egg yolk, pepper, cream cheese, and flour
7) Mash the dough with your hands, until you have a workable mixture
8) Shape the gnocchi using your hands
9) Bake the gnocchi in the air fryer at 250F for 4 minutes
10) In a small saucepan melt the butter
11) Serve the gnocchi with the melted butter

ITALIAN-STYLE PORK TENDERLOINS

PREPARATION TIME: 15 MINUTES- **COOKING TIME:** 30 MINUTES- **SERVINGS:** 4

CALORIES: 77, **CARBOHYDRATES:** 2g, **PROTEINS:** 5g, **FAT:** 1g

INGREDIENTS
1 cup Parmesan cheese
2 tablespoons olive oil
3 cloves of garlic
4 pork tenderloins
Salt and pepper to taste
A pinch of rosemary

DIRECTIONS
1) Preheat the air fryer to 350F
2) In a bowl, mix the olive oil, garlic, rosemary, salt, and pepper
3) Spread the mixture on the pork tenderloins
4) Bake the fillets at 350F for 25 minutes
5) Finish the fillets with the Parmesan cheese
6) Let them air fry for another 5 minutes, taking care that the cheese does not burn
7) Let the fillets rest for 5 minutes
8) Serve them with some vegetables

LAMB CHOPS

PREPARATION TIME: 190 MINUTES- **COOKING TIME:** 16 MINUTES- **SERVINGS: 4**

CALORIES: 162, **CARBOHYDRATES:** 1g, **PROTEINS:** 15g, **FAT:** 4g

INGREDIENTS
- 1 tablespoon paprika
- 1 tablespoon smoked paprika
- 1 pinch of garlic powder
- 2 tablespoons olive oil
- 5 lamb chops
- Salt and pepper to taste
- A pinch of oregano

DIRECTIONS
1) Mix paprika, smoked paprika, oregano, garlic, and olive oil in a bowl
2) Sprinkle the ribs with the freshly prepared mixture
3) Place them in the refrigerator for 3 hours
4) After 3 hours, bake the ribs in the air fryer at 350F for 16 minutes, turning them halfway through cooking
5) Serve the ribs freshly cooked

LEMON LAMB STEAKS

PREPARATION TIME: 15 MINUTES- **COOKING TIME:** 7 MINUTES- **SERVINGS:** 4

CALORIES: 98, **CARBOHYDRATES:** 1g, **PROTEINS:** 8g, **FAT:** 5g

INGREDIENTS
- 1 pinch of oregano
- 1 pinch rosemary
- 1 pinch of thyme
- 3 cups sliced lamb meat
- 2 tablespoons olive oil
- 2 teaspoons lemon juice
- A pinch of salt

DIRECTIONS
1) Preheat the air fryer to 350F
2) Season the steaks with spices
3) Let them rest for a few minutes so they can absorb all the flavors
4) Air fry the steaks at 350F for 7 minutes, turning them in the middle of cooking
5) Serve them freshly cooked

MEATBALLS

PREPARATION TIME: 15 MINUTES- **COOKING TIME:** 11 MINUTES- **SERVINGS:** 4

CALORIES: 88, **CARBOHYDRATES:** 3g, **PROTEINS:** 8g, **FAT:** 3g

INGREDIENTS
- 1 onion
- 1 egg
- ½ pound minced meat
- 3 cups minced garlic
- 1/2 cup Parmesan cheese
- Pepper to taste
- Parsley to taste
- Salt to taste

DIRECTIONS
1) Combine all the ingredients in a bowl
2) Mix until smooth
3) Using your hands, make meatballs from the mixture
4) Bake the meatballs in the air fryer at 350F for 11 minutes.
5) Serve them accompanied by vegetables or potatoes

MOZZARELLA CROSTONE WITH CHICKEN AND PEPPERS

PREPARATION TIME: 10 MINUTES- **COOKING TIME:** 15 MINUTES- **SERVINGS:** 4

CALORIES: 153, **CARBOHYDRATES:** 5g, **PROTEINS:** 14g, **FAT:** 4g

INGREDIENTS
- 1 tablespoon olive oil
- 4.5oz mozzarella cheese
- 2 cups chopped bell peppers
- 2 cups chicken cut into cubes
- 0.5oz of Parmesan cheese
- A pinch of pepper
- A pinch of salt

DIRECTIONS
1) In a bowl, mix chicken with peppers, salt, pepper, and olive oil
2) Add the sliced mozzarella cheese
3) Air fry everything at 350F for 15 minutes or until the mozzarella forms a nice crust
4) Serve immediately with a sprinkling of Parmesan cheese

ORIENTAL-STYLE SPICED LAMB

PREPARATION TIME: 130 MINUTES- **COOKING TIME:** 10 MINUTES- **SERVINGS:** 4

CALORIES: 129, **CARBOHYDRATES:** 2g, **PROTEINS:** 6g, **FAT:** 2g

INGREDIENTS
- 1 tablespoon soy sauce
- 2 tablespoons seed oil
- 2 finely chopped red peppers
- 4 lamb steaks
- A pinch of cayenne
- A pinch of cumin
- A pinch of pepper
- A pinch of salt
- One clove of minced garlic

DIRECTIONS
1) In a bowl, mix the cumin and cayenne
2) Toss the steaks in the freshly prepared spice mix
3) Add the peppers, oil, soy sauce, garlic, salt, and pepper
4) Mix well
5) Let stand in the refrigerator for a couple of hours
6) Air fry the meat at 350F for 10 minutes
7) Serve the steaks freshly cooked

PAPRIKA BACON CUBES

PREPARATION TIME: 5 MINUTES- **COOKING TIME:** 20 MINUTES- **SERVINGS:** 4

CALORIES: 139, **CARBOHYDRATES:** 1g, **PROTEINS:** 13g, **FAT:** 2g

INGREDIENTS
- Two tablespoons of olive oil
- Half a pound of diced bacon
- Salt and pepper to taste
- A pinch of paprika

DIRECTIONS
1) In a bowl, place the paprika, oil, salt, and pepper
2) Pass the bacon cubes through the mixture
3) Air fry the bacon cubes at 250F for 20 minutes, stirring them halfway through cooking

PAPRIKA PORK RIBS

PREPARATION TIME: 10 MINUTES- **COOKING TIME:** 20 MINUTES- **SERVINGS: 4**

CALORIES: 112, **CARBOHYDRATES:** 5g, **PROTEINS:** 5g, **FAT:** 3g

INGREDIENTS
- 1 tablespoon salt
- 3 cups pork ribs from your local butcher's shop
- 2 tablespoons paprika
- 3 tablespoons olive oil

DIRECTIONS
1) In a bowl, mix with your hands the pork ribs, paprika, salt, and olive oil
2) Keep stirring until the ribs are full of seasoning
3) Air fry the ribs at 350F for 20 minutes
4) They will be ready as soon as the meat comes off the bone with ease
5) Serve them with some potatoes or vegetables

PARMESAN TROUT

PREPARATION TIME: 15 MINUTES- **COOKING TIME:** 5 MINUTES- **SERVINGS: 4**

CALORIES: 154, **CARBOHYDRATES:** 2g, **PROTEINS:** 11g, **FAT:** 3g

INGREDIENTS
- 1 cup almond flour
- 2 eggs
- 1.5lbs trout fillets
- 1/2 cup Parmesan cheese
- Lemon zest as much as needed
- A pinch of pepper
- A pinch of salt
- One clove of minced garlic

DIRECTIONS
1) In a bowl, beat the eggs
2) In another bowl, mix the Parmesan cheese, lemon zest, salt, pepper, and garlic
3) Pat the trout dry with paper towel
4) Sprinkle the fillets with flour, making sure they are coated on both sides
5) Dip the fillets in the egg
6) Dip the fillets in the mixture with the Parmesan cheese and spices
7) Air fry the fillets at 400F for 5 minutes, until the Parmesan cheese has melted, forming a golden crust
8) Serve the fillets freshly cooked

PLAIN STEAK

PREPARATION TIME: 5 MINUTES- **COOKING TIME:** 14 MINUTES- **SERVINGS:** 4

CALORIES: 88, CARBOHYDRATES: 0g, PROTEINS: 13g, FAT: 7g

INGREDIENTS	DIRECTIONS
2 pork steaks A pinch of pepper A pinch of salt	1) Coat the steaks with salt and pepper 2) Bake them at 350F for 14 minutes, remembering to turn them halfway through cooking 3) Serve them with vegetables or potatoes

PORK CHOPS WITH 4 KINDS OF CHEESE

PREPARATION TIME: 20 MINUTES- **COOKING TIME:** 20 MINUTES- **SERVINGS:** 4

CALORIES: 156, CARBOHYDRATES: 5g, PROTEINS: 18g, FAT: 4g

INGREDIENTS	DIRECTIONS
4 pork chops 1/2 cup cream cheese 1/2 cup gorgonzola 1/2 cup mozzarella 1/2 cup Parmesan cheese	1) In a saucepan, melt the gorgonzola cheese 2) Add the other cheeses 3) Over low heat, continue stirring until a smooth sauce is created 4) Air fry the pork chops at 350F for 20 minutes 5) Serve the pork chops with the 4-cheese sauce

PORK RIBS WITH PARMESAN CHEESE

PREPARATION TIME: 15 MINUTES- **COOKING TIME:** 15 MINUTES- **SERVINGS:** 4

CALORIES: 179, CARBOHYDRATES: 3g, PROTEINS: 5g, FAT: 4g

INGREDIENTS	DIRECTIONS
3/4 cup Parmesan cheese 2 eggs 6 pork chops A tablespoon of paprika A pinch of onion A pinch of pepper A pinch of chili pepper A pinch of salt	1) Preheat the air fryer to 400F 2) In a bowl, beat the eggs 3) On a plate, put the rest of the ingredients except the meat 4) Dip the ribs in the eggs 5) Pass the ribs in the dish with the spices and Parmesan cheese 6) Air fry the ribs for 15 minutes, turning them halfway through cooking 7) Serve them freshly cooked

SALMON FILLETS IN WALNUT CRUST

PREPARATION TIME: 10 MINUTES - **COOKING TIME:** 12 MINUTES - **SERVINGS: 4**

CALORIES: 63, **CARBOHYDRATES:** 1g, **PROTEINS:** 7g, **FAT:** 1g

INGREDIENTS

- 1 cup finely chopped walnuts
- 4 salmon fillets
- One tablespoon of olive oil
- A pinch of fresh oregano
- A pinch of pepper
- A pinch of salt

DIRECTIONS

1) Preheat the air fryer to 400F
2) In a bowl, add and mix the oil, salt, pepper, and walnuts
3) Toss the salmon in the spices
4) Air fry the salmon for 12 minutes, turning halfway through cooking
5) Sprinkle the salmon with oregano
6) Serve it freshly cooked

TROUT WITH GARLIC AND LEMON

PREPARATION TIME: 10 MINUTES - **COOKING TIME:** 10 MINUTES - **SERVINGS: 4**

CALORIES: 56, **CARBOHYDRATES:** 2g, **PROTEINS:** 9g, **FAT:** 1g

INGREDIENTS

- 1.75lbs trout fillets
- 4 lemon wedges
- Pepper to taste
- Salt to taste
- One tablespoon of olive oil
- A dash of lemon juice
- A pinch of fresh parsley
- A pinch of garlic powder

DIRECTIONS

1) Preheat the air fryer to 350F
2) Pat the trout fillets dry with paper towel
3) Sprinkle the fillets with olive oil, garlic powder, lemon, salt, and pepper
4) Bake the fillets in the air fryer at 350F for 10 minutes, turning them halfway through cooking
5) Finish them with parsley
6) Serve them accompanied by a lemon wedge

SESAME PORK RIBS

PREPARATION TIME: 30 MINUTES- **COOKING TIME:** 20 MINUTES- **SERVINGS:** 4

CALORIES: 119, **CARBOHYDRATES:** 1g, **PROTEINS:** 23g, **FAT:** 6g

INGREDIENTS
- 3 cups of ribs from your local butcher's shop
- 2 tablespoons apple cider vinegar
- 2 tablespoons honey
- 2 tablespoons seed oil
- 2 drops of liquid stevia
- 2 cloves of garlic
- 1/2 cup soy sauce
- 1/4 cup cold water

DIRECTIONS
1) To prepare the sauce, in a bowl combine the soy sauce, vinegar, honey, oil, liquid stevia, and garlic
2) Stir well
3) Cook over low heat for a few minutes
4) Add the water to the sauce
5) Keep stirring until the mixture is smooth
6) Cut the ribs into pieces so they fit in the air fryer
7) Drizzle the ribs with the sauce you just prepared
8) Air fry the ribs at 350F for 20 minutes, turning them halfway through cooking
9) Let the ribs rest for a few minutes
10) Serve them with some vegetables of your taste

SMOKED STEAKS

PREPARATION TIME: 125 MINUTES- **COOKING TIME:** 10 MINUTES- **SERVINGS:** 4

CALORIES: 156, **CARBOHYDRATES:** 1g, **PROTEINS:** 12g, **FAT:** 3g

INGREDIENTS
- 1 teaspoon soy sauce
- 1 tablespoon smoked sauce
- 2 beef steaks
- A pinch of pepper
- A pinch of salt

DIRECTIONS
1) In a bowl, add all the ingredients, making sure the steaks are well coated
2) Let rest in the refrigerator for two hours
3) Air fry the steaks in the air fryer at 350F for 10 minutes, turning them after 5 minutes
4) Serve them freshly cooked

SPICE MARINATED CHICKEN

PREPARATION TIME: 200 MINUTES- **COOKING TIME:** 12 MINUTES- **SERVINGS: 4**

CALORIES: 165, **CARBOHYDRATES:** 5g, **PROTEINS:** 5g, **FAT:** 8g

INGREDIENTS
- 1/2 cup red wine
- 3 chicken steaks
- One tablespoon of hot sauce
- A pinch of pepper
- A pinch of salt
- One clove of minced garlic

DIRECTIONS
1) In a bowl, combine the chicken, garlic, red wine, hot sauce, salt, and pepper
2) Let stand in the refrigerator for 3 hours
3) Drain the steaks
4) Air fry them at 350F for 12 minutes, turning them halfway through cooking
5) Serve freshly cooked

SPICED PORK STEAKS

PREPARATION TIME: 5 MINUTES- **COOKING TIME:** 10 MINUTES- **SERVINGS: 4**

CALORIES: 174, **CARBOHYDRATES:** 3g, **PROTEINS:** 12g, **FAT:** 1g

INGREDIENTS
- 1 tablespoon olive oil
- 4 pork steaks
- A pinch of pepper
- A pinch of salt
- A handful of oregano
- One clove of minced garlic

DIRECTIONS
1) Preheat the air fryer to 350F
2) In a bowl, mix the garlic, olive oil, oregano, pepper, and salt
3) Spread the sauce over the pork steaks
4) Air fry the steaks for 10 minutes
5) Serve them freshly cooked

SWEET-AND-SOUR PORK STEAKS

PREPARATION TIME: 30 MINUTES- **COOKING TIME:** 6 MINUTES- **SERVINGS:** 4

CALORIES: 112, **CARBOHYDRATES:** 3g, **PROTEINS:** 8g, **FAT:** 2g

INGREDIENTS

For the sauce:
- 1 tablespoon olive oil
- 1 tablespoon soy sauce
- 1 red bell pepper cut into slices
- 1 sliced green bell pepper
- 2 drops of liquid liquid stevia
- 1/2 cup rice vinegar
- 1 cup sugar-free orange juice
- Half a chopped onion

For the steaks:
- 1 tablespoon olive oil
- 3 eggs
- 4 pork steaks
- A pinch of pepper
- A pinch of salt

DIRECTIONS

1) In a bowl, mix the orange juice, vinegar, liquid stevia, and soy sauce until smooth
2) In a small frying pan, heat oil
3) Add peppers and onion
4) Stir for 2 to 3 minutes, until peppers are slightly crispy
5) Add sauce prepared earlier
6) Continue stirring until sauce is reduced
7) Remove sauce from heat and let it rest for 5 minutes
8) In a bowl, stir in the spices
9) In another bowl, add the eggs and oil
10) Mash each steak in the egg and oil mixture
11) Pass each steak through the spices
12) Air fry the steaks at 350F for 4 minutes
13) Turn them over and air fry them for 2 more minutes
14) Serve them freshly cooked with the sweet and sour sauce

THYME AND MUSHROOMS MEATLOAF

PREPARATION TIME: 10 MINUTES- **COOKING TIME:** 25 MINUTES- **SERVINGS:** 4

CALORIES: 109, **CARBOHYDRATES:** g, **PROTEINS:** 13g, **FAT:** 2g

INGREDIENTS
- 1 chopped onion
- 1 egg
- 1 cup chopped porcini mushrooms
- 3 cups beef
- 2 cups almond flour
- A pinch of pepper

DIRECTIONS

1) Mix all the ingredients in a bowl until smooth
2) Transfer the mixture to the air fryer
3) Cover it with foil
4) Bake the meatloaf at 400F for 25 minutes
5) Serve the meatloaf freshly cooked

TUNA STEAK WITH RED ONIONS

PREPARATION TIME: 10 MINUTES- **COOKING TIME:** 10 MINUTES- **SERVINGS:** 4

CALORIES: 99, **CARBOHYDRATES:** 7g, **PROTEINS:** 8g, **FAT:** 2g

INGREDIENTS
- 1 lemon cut into wedges
- 3/4 cup finely chopped red onion
- 4 tuna fillets
- A pinch of pepper
- A pinch of rosemary
- A pinch of salt

DIRECTIONS
1) Preheat the air fryer to 400F
2) Place the tuna in the air fryer and top with the red onions
3) Add the olive oil, salt, pepper, and rosemary
4) Bake the tuna for 10 minutes, turning it halfway through cooking
5) Serve it with a lemon wedge

TURMERIC-ORANGE MARINATED STEAK

PREPARATION TIME: 150 MINUTES- **COOKING TIME:** 15 MINUTES- **SERVINGS:** 4

CALORIES: 168, **CARBOHYDRATES:** 1g, **PROTEINS:** 19g, **FAT:** 3g

INGREDIENTS
- 1 teaspoon turmeric
- 2 tablespoons olive oil
- 2 tablespoons lime juice
- 4 beef steaks
- 4 cloves of garlic
- 1/4 cup orange juice
- Salt and pepper to taste

DIRECTIONS
1) Add all the ingredients to a bowl
2) Let steaks marinate for a couple of hours
3) Preheat the air fryer to 350F
4) Bake the steaks for 15 minutes, turning them halfway through cooking
5) Let the steaks rest for 10 minutes so that the flavors penetrate the meat even better
6) Serve the steaks with vegetables

WESTERN-STYLE PORK LOIN

PREPARATION TIME: 50 MINUTES- **COOKING TIME:** 40 MINUTES- **SERVINGS:** 4

CALORIES: 140, **CARBOHYDRATES:** 2g, **PROTEINS:** 13g, **FAT:** 7g

INGREDIENTS
- 1 cup chopped onion
- 2 jalapenos chilies
- 1/2 cup seed oil
- 3 cups pork loin
- A pinch of turmeric
- A pinch of pepper
- A pinch of salt
- A pinch of minced garlic

DIRECTIONS
1) In a bowl, put the oil, onions, jalapenos, turmeric, salt, pepper, and garlic
2) Mix well
3) Pass the meat through the bowl
4) Let it rest for 30 minutes so that it absorbs the flavors well
5) Bake the meat in the air fryer at 350F for 40 minutes
6) Let the meat rest for 10 minutes after cooking

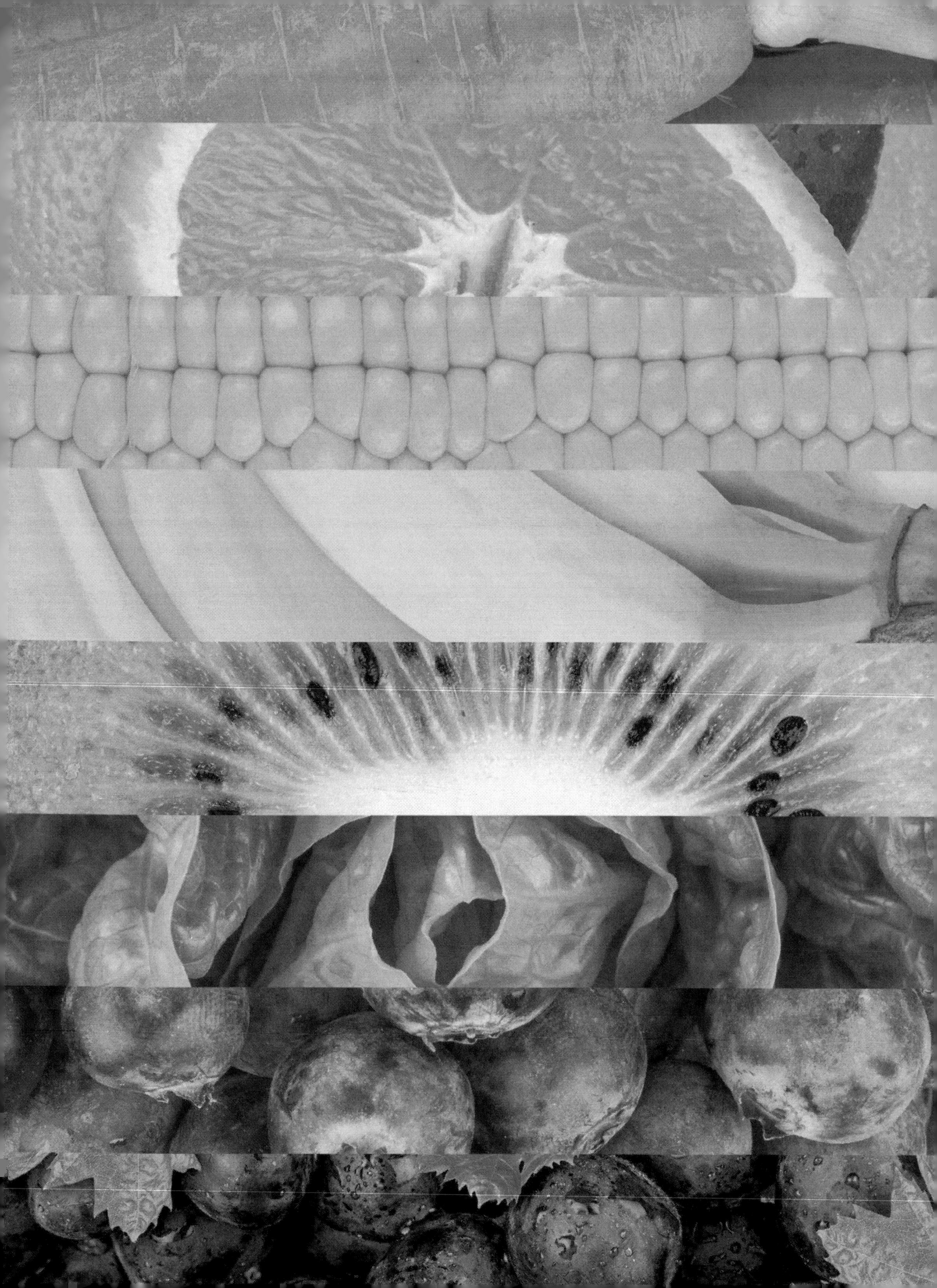

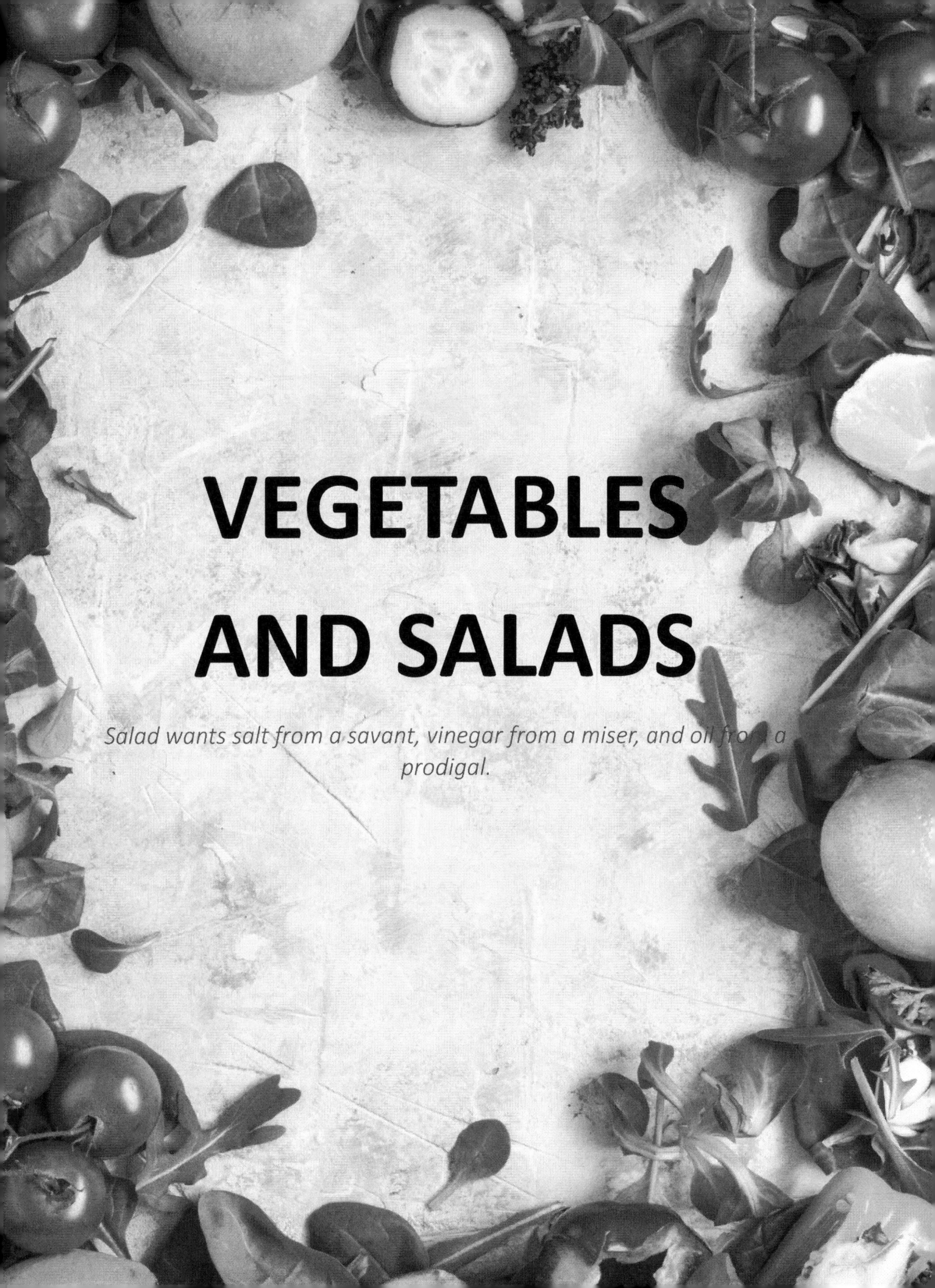

VEGETABLES AND SALADS

Salad wants salt from a savant, vinegar from a miser, and oil from a prodigal.

AVOCADO EGGS

PREPARATION TIME: 10 MINUTES- **COOKING TIME:** 15 MINUTES- **SERVINGS:** 4

CALORIES: 98, **CARBOHYDRATES:** 4g, **PROTEINS:** 7g, **FAT:** 2g

INGREDIENTS	DIRECTIONS
1 avocado 2 eggs 0.5oz butter A pinch of turmeric A pinch of pepper A pinch of salt	1) Mix turmeric, pepper, and salt in a bowl 2) Cut the avocado into two pieces 3) In another bowl, crack the eggs open 4) Sprinkle the eggs with the spices 5) Put the eggs in the avocado halves 6) Bake the avocado in the air fryer at 350F for 15 minutes 7) Serve freshly cooked

BELL PEPPER SALAD

PREPARATION TIME: 5 MINUTES- **COOKING TIME:** 12 MINUTES- **SERVINGS:** 4

CALORIES: 98, **CARBOHYDRATES:** 3g, **PROTEINS:** 6g, **FAT:** 2g

INGREDIENTS	DIRECTIONS
1 red onion cut into small pieces 1 red bell pepper chopped into small pieces 1 green bell pepper cut into small pieces 1 zucchini cut into small pieces 1 cup porcini mushrooms 1 cup pitted olives 2 cups cherry tomatoes	1) In a bowl, mix the zucchini with the mushrooms, peppers, onion, salt, and oil 2) Bake in the air fryer at 200F for 12 minutes 3) In a bowl, mix the cooked vegetables with the other vegetables 4) Serve freshly cooked

CORN AND TOMATO SALAD

PREPARATION TIME: 5 MINUTES- **COOKING TIME:** 10 MINUTES- **SERVINGS:** 4

CALORIES: 103, **CARBOHYDRATES:** 7g, **PROTEINS:** 6g, **FAT:** 6g

INGREDIENTS	DIRECTIONS
1 onion, chopped 1 tablespoon olive oil 2 cups iceberg lettuce 12 sliced cherry tomatoes 3 cups corn Salt and pepper to taste	1) Put the corn in the air fryer 2) Add the oil, salt, and pepper 3) Bake at 350F for 10 minutes 4) Put the corn in a bowl 5) Add the iceberg lettuce and serve freshly cooked

CREAMY ZUCCHINI AND POTATOES

PREPARATION TIME: 15 MINUTES- **COOKING TIME:** 14 MINUTES- **SERVINGS: 4**

CALORIES: 133, **CARBOHYDRATES:** 5g, **PROTEINS:** 15g, **FAT:** 3g

INGREDIENTS
- 2 chopped onions
- 2 tablespoons olive
- 2 sweet potatoes peeled and cut into wedges
- 1 cup coconut milk
- 3 zucchini
- Salt and pepper to taste
- A pinch of basil
- A pinch of rosemary

DIRECTIONS
1) In a skillet, cook the onions and oil for a couple of minutes
2) Add the rest of the ingredients
3) Continue stirring for 5 minutes
4) Pour everything into the air fryer
5) Bake at 350F for 14 minutes, stirring often
6) Serve freshly cooked

CRISPY BROCCOLI SALAD

PREPARATION TIME: 5 MINUTES- **COOKING TIME:** 7 MINUTES- **SERVINGS: 4**

CALORIES: 102, **CARBOHYDRATES:** 6g, **PROTEINS:** 4g, **FAT:** 7g

INGREDIENTS
- 1 tablespoon olive oil
- 0.5oz lemon juice
- 1/2 cup of broccoli
- 1/2 cup almonds
- 1/2 cup Parmesan cheese
- A pinch of pepper
- A pinch of salt

DIRECTIONS
1) In a bowl, mix broccoli with olive oil
2) Sprinkle the broccoli with salt, pepper, and the lemon juice
3) Bake the broccoli in the air fryer at 350F for 7 minutes, stirring halfway through
4) Serve the broccoli freshly cooked, finishing it off with Parmesan cheese

CRUNCHY GREEN BEANS

PREPARATION TIME: 10 MINUTES- **COOKING TIME:** 7 MINUTES- **SERVINGS: 4**

CALORIES: 93, **CARBOHYDRATES:** 4g, **PROTEINS:** 6g, **FAT:** 4g

INGREDIENTS
- 1 egg
- 2 tablespoons oil
- 1/2 cup green beans
- 1/2 cup Parmesan cheese
- A pinch of pepper
- A pinch of salt
- A pinch of crushed red pepper

DIRECTIONS
1) In a bowl, combine the green beans, eggs, Parmesan cheese, salt, and red pepper
2) Mix well and then add the oil
3) Air fry at 350F for 4 minutes
4) Stir it and cook for another 3 minutes
5) Serve them freshly cooked

EGGS AND TOMATOES

PREPARATION TIME: 5 MINUTES- **COOKING TIME:** 9 MINUTES- **SERVINGS:** 4

CALORIES: 100, **CARBOHYDRATES:** 2g, **PROTEINS:** 7g, **FAT:** 1g

INGREDIENTS
- 1/2 cup milk
- 4 eggs
- 1/2 cup Parmesan cheese
- 8 cherry tomatoes
- Salt and pepper to taste

DIRECTIONS
1) Preheat the air fryer to 400F
2) In a bowl, mix the eggs, Parmesan cheese, salt, and pepper
3) Pour into the air fryer
4) Bake for 6 minutes
5) Add tomatoes and cook for another 3 minutes
6) Serve freshly cooked

HERB LENTILS

PREPARATION TIME: 5 MINUTES- **COOKING TIME:** 15 MINUTES- **SERVINGS:** 4

CALORIES: 96, **CARBOHYDRATES:** 2g, **PROTEINS:** 4g, **FAT:** 2g

INGREDIENTS
- 1/2 cup chopped onion
- 2 tablespoons olive oil
- 2 cups of lentils
- 2 cups finely chopped spinach

DIRECTIONS
1) In the air fryer put all the ingredients
2) Bake at 400F for 15 minutes
3) Serve freshly cooked

LEEK SALAD

PREPARATION TIME: 5 MINUTES- **COOKING TIME:** 12 MINUTES- **SERVINGS:** 4

CALORIES: 31, **CARBOHYDRATES:** 3g, **PROTEINS:** 6g, **FAT:** 1g

INGREDIENTS
- 1 tablespoon cumin
- 1 clove of garlic, minced
- 6 leeks cut into pieces
- Salt and pepper to taste
- 1 tablespoon of olive oil

DIRECTIONS
1) In a baking dish combine all the ingredients
2) Mix well
3) Bake in the air fryer at 350F for 12 minutes
4) Serve freshly cooked

OREGANO PEPPERS

PREPARATION TIME: 5 MINUTES- **COOKING TIME:** 14 MINUTES- **SERVINGS:** 4

CALORIES: 72, **CARBOHYDRATES:** 3g, **PROTEINS:** 7g, **FAT:** 2g

INGREDIENTS	DIRECTIONS
1 onion, chopped 1 tablespoon olive oil 1 chopped yellow bell pepper 1 chopped red bell pepper 1 chopped green bell pepper 1 cup cheese of your choice Salt and pepper to taste	1) In the air fryer put all the ingredients except the cheese 2) Mix well 3) Bake at 350F for 10 minutes, stirring often 4) Add cheese and cook for another 4 minutes 5) Serve freshly cooked

ORIENTAL-STYLE ASPARAGUS

PREPARATION TIME: 5 MINUTES- **COOKING TIME:** 10 MINUTES- **SERVINGS:** 4

CALORIES: 70, **CARBOHYDRATES:** 7g, **PROTEINS:** 3g, **FAT:** 3g

INGREDIENTS	DIRECTIONS
1 tablespoon olive oil 4 asparagus pieces 4 cloves of garlic, minced Salt and pepper to taste	1) In the air fryer put all the ingredients 2) Bake at 350F for 10 minutes 3) Serve freshly cooked

SPINACH SALAD

PREPARATION TIME: 5 MINUTES- **COOKING TIME:** 10 MINUTES- **SERVINGS:** 4

CALORIES: 60, **CARBOHYDRATES:** 4g, **PROTEINS:** 6g, **FAT:** 3g

INGREDIENTS	DIRECTIONS
2 1/2 cups spinach 1/4 cup apple cider vinegar A pinch of pepper A pinch of salt	1) Combine all the ingredients in the air fryer 2) Mix well 3) Bake at 350F for 10 minutes 4) Serve the spinach freshly cooked

ZUCCHINI SALAD

PREPARATION TIME: 5 MINUTES- **COOKING TIME**: 10 MINUTES- **SERVINGS**: 4

CALORIES: 70, **CARBOHYDRATES**: 2g, **PROTEINS**: 6g, **FAT**: 4g

INGREDIENTS
1 zucchini peeled and diced
2 tablespoons olive oil
1/2 cup coconut cream
1/2 cup diced carrots
A pinch of pepper
A pinch of salt

DIRECTIONS
1) In a baking dish, combine all the ingredients
2) Mix them well
3) Bake in the air fryer at 400F for 10 minutes, turning often
4) Serve freshly cooked

SNACKS

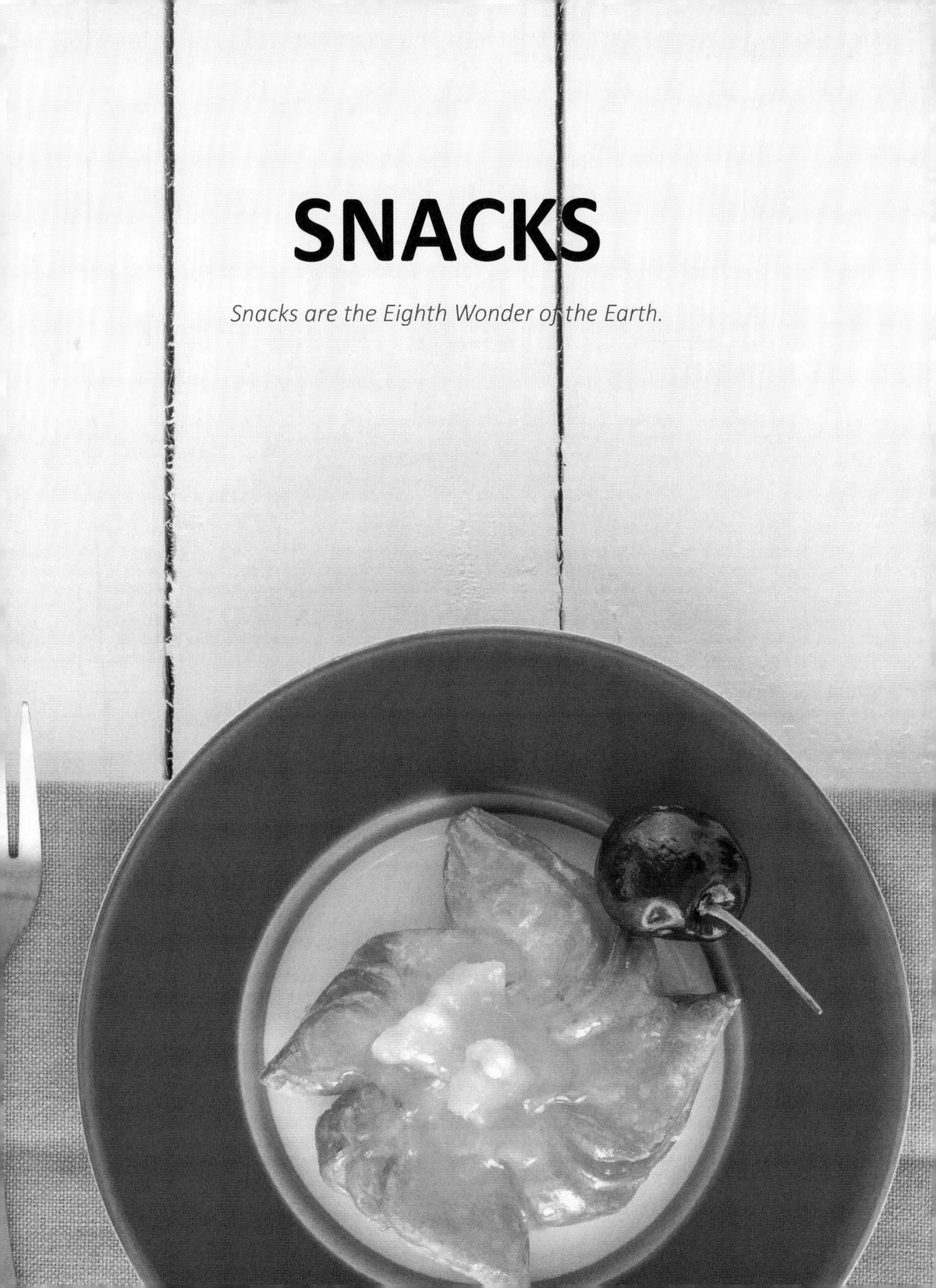

Snacks are the Eighth Wonder of the Earth.

ALMOND SANDWICHES

PREPARATION TIME: 15 MINUTES- **COOKING TIME:** 13 MINUTES- **SERVINGS: 4**

CALORIES: 72, **CARBOHYDRATES:** 2g, **PROTEINS:** 3g, **FAT:** 5g

INGREDIENTS
- 2 tablespoons of baking powder
- 1 teaspoon apple cider vinegar
- 2 drops of liquid stevia
- 1/2 cup warm water
- 2 cups almond flour
- 4 eggs
- A pinch of salt

DIRECTIONS
1) In a bowl, put the almond flour, baking powder, and salt
2) In another bowl, crack open the eggs
3) Beat the eggs
4) Add the liquid stevia and apple cider vinegar
5) Add the hot water to the bowl with the flour
6) Stirring, add the mixture with the eggs
7) Mix well until the mixture is firm and homogeneous
8) Preheat the air fryer to 350F
9) Using your hands, divide the dough into 10 small buns
10) Bake each bun for 13 minutes
11) Let the buns rest and serve them at room temperature

AVOCADO STICKS

PREPARATION TIME: 10 MINUTES- **COOKING TIME:** 14 MINUTES- **SERVINGS: 4**

CALORIES: 131g, **CARBOHYDRATES:** 4g, **PROTEINS:** 2, **FAT:** 4g

INGREDIENTS
- 1 avocado, pitted and cut in half
- 1 tablespoon coconut flakes
- 1 egg

DIRECTIONS
1) Cut the avocado into four parts
2) Dip the avocado in the egg
3) Sprinkle the avocado with coconut flakes
4) Bake the avocado in the air fryer at 350F for 7 minutes per side
5) Serve the avocado sticks at room temperature

BACON-WRAPPED AVOCADO

PREPARATION TIME: 20 MINUTES- **COOKING TIME:** 10 MINUTES- **SERVINGS: 4**

CALORIES: 116, **CARBOHYDRATES:** 5g, **PROTEINS:** 8g, **FAT:** 6g

INGREDIENTS

- 1 tablespoon flaked coconut
- 1 tablespoon olive oil
- 1 egg
- 2 pitted avocados
- 3 slices of bacon
- A pinch of pepper
- A pinch of rosemary
- A pinch of salt

DIRECTIONS

1) Peel the avocados and cut them into 8 parts
2) In a bowl, beat the eggs
3) Add the coconut flakes, salt, pepper, oil, and rosemary
4) Dip the avocado slices in the mixture
5) Roll each avocado slice in a slice of bacon
6) Air fry at 350F for 10 minutes, turning halfway through cooking
7) Serve freshly cooked

BLUEBERRY PUDDING

PREPARATION TIME: 25 MINUTES- **COOKING TIME:** 25 MINUTES- **SERVINGS: 4**

CALORIES: 150, **CARBOHYDRATES:** 7g, **PROTEINS:** 4g, **FAT:** 3g

INGREDIENTS

- 1/2 cup oats
- 1/2 cup almond flour
- 2 3/4 cups blueberries
- 1/2 cup butter
- 1/2 cup maple syrup

DIRECTIONS

1) Using a food processor, mix oats with the flour, butter, and maple syrup
2) Melt the butter on a baking sheet
3) Arrange the blueberries on top
4) Pour the previously prepared mixture over the blueberries
5) Bake in the air fryer at 350F for 25 minutes
6) Pour the mixture into special cups
7) Let cool and serve at room temperature

BREADED ZUCCHINI CHIPS

PREPARATION TIME: 10 MINUTES - **COOKING TIME:** 12 MINUTES - **SERVINGS:** 4

CALORIES: 107, **CARBOHYDRATES:** 19g, **PROTEINS:** 3g, **FAT:** 2g

INGREDIENTS
1 steamed and mashed potato
2 tablespoons of almond flour
2 tablespoons olive oil
2 cloves of garlic, minced
2 zucchini, peeled

DIRECTIONS
1) Preheat the air fryer to 350F
2) Mix all the ingredients in a bowl
3) Using your hands, form fairly thin medallions with the resulting mixture
4) Bake for 12 minutes, turning the medallions often
5) Serve them with a drizzle of mayonnaise or sauce of your choice

BRUSSELS SPROUTS WITH THYME AND PARSLEY

PREPARATION TIME: 5 MINUTES - **COOKING TIME:** 20 MINUTES - **SERVINGS:** 4

CALORIES: 79, **CARBOHYDRATES:** 8g, **PROTEINS:** 4g, **FAT:** 2g

INGREDIENTS
1 pinch of parsley
2 1/2 cups of Brussels sprouts
One tablespoon of seed oil
A pinch of salt

DIRECTIONS
1) Mix all the ingredients in a bowl
2) Air fry the sprouts at 400F for 20 minutes
3) Serve them freshly cooked

CALAMARI RINGS WITH ALMONDS

PREPARATION TIME: 20 MINUTES - **COOKING TIME:** 8 MINUTES - **SERVINGS:** 4

CALORIES: **CARBOHYDRATES:** 3g, **PROTEINS:** 14g, **FAT:** 2g

INGREDIENTS
1 teaspoon lemon juice
1 egg
2 cups almond flour
3 cups calamari
Lemon zest to taste
A pinch of pepper
A pinch of salt

DIRECTIONS
1) Wash and peel the calamari
2) Cut the calamari into small rings
3) Beat the egg in a bowl
4) Add the lemon zest, salt, and pepper to the egg, continuing to mix
5) Drizzle the calamari rings with lemon juice
6) Put the calamari in the egg and mix well
7) Let them sit for 5 minutes
8) Dip the calamari in the almond flour
9) Air fry the calamari at 350F for 8 minutes

CAULIFLOWER AND CHEESE GNOCCHI

PREPARATION TIME: 25 MINUTES- **COOKING TIME:** 8 MINUTES- **SERVINGS:** 4

CALORIES: 152, **CARBOHYDRATES:** 1g, **PROTEINS:** 9g, **FAT:** 12g

INGREDIENTS

- 1 tablespoon of seed oil
- 1 cup cheese of your choice
- 2 cups boiled and finely chopped cauliflower
- 1/2 cup cream cheese
- A pinch of garlic powder
- A pinch of salt

DIRECTIONS

1) Using a food processor, chop the cauliflower along with the garlic powder, cream cheese, cheese of your choice, and salt
2) Form the gnocchi with your hands
3) Place them in the refrigerator for 10 minutes
4) Bake the gnocchi in the air fryer at 350F for 8 minutes, turning them halfway through
5) Serve them freshly cooked with a sprinkling of Parmesan cheese

CHEESE AND BACON BROCCOLI

PREPARATION TIME: 5 MINUTES- **COOKING TIME:** 10 MINUTES- **SERVINGS:** 4

CALORIES: 161, **CARBOHYDRATES:** 1g, **PROTEINS:** 18g, **FAT:** 5g

INGREDIENTS

- 1 tablespoon olive oil
- 1 shallot, finely chopped
- 1 cup cheese of your choice
- 1/2 cup fresh broccoli
- 4 slices of toasted and crispy bacon

DIRECTIONS

1) Put the broccoli in the air fryer and sprinkle them with oil
2) Bake them at 350F for 10 minutes
3) While cooking, stir them two or three times to prevent them from burning
4) Once ready, sprinkle the broccoli with cheese
5) Serve them on a slice of bacon

CHEESE FRIED ZUCCHINI

PREPARATION TIME: 10 MINUTES- **COOKING TIME:** 7 MINUTES- **SERVINGS:** 4

CALORIES: 133, **CARBOHYDRATES:** 3g, **PROTEINS:** 9g, **FAT:** 9g

INGREDIENTS
1 tablespoon almond flour
1 tablespoon coconut flour
1 mozzarella cheese
1 zucchini
0.5oz butter
1/2 cup cheese of your choice
A pinch of salt

DIRECTIONS
1) In a bowl, cut the mozzarella and cheese
2) Combine the cheese and zucchini
3) Add the flours
4) Mix well
5) Let it marinate for 3 minutes
6) Air fry at 350F for 5 minutes
7) Sprinkle the zucchini with butter
8) Cook for 2 more minutes
9) Serve freshly cooked with a pinch of salt

CHEESE STICKS

PREPARATION TIME: 15 MINUTES- **COOKING TIME:** 10 MINUTES- **SERVINGS:** 4

CALORIES: 62, **CARBOHYDRATES:** 2g, **PROTEINS:** 4g, **FAT:** 4g

INGREDIENTS
1 egg
1 cup Parmesan cheese
1/2 cup almond flour
A piece of cheese of your choice, cut into 8 thin rectangles
A pinch of garlic powder
A pinch of rosemary

DIRECTIONS
1) Beat the egg in a bowl
2) Add the flour, Parmesan cheese, garlic, and rosemary
3) Continue stirring until smooth
4) Dip the cheese pieces into the resulting sauce
5) Cook the cheese sticks in the air fryer at 350F for 10 minutes
6) Serve them freshly cooked

CHEESE CAULIFLOWER

PREPARATION TIME: 5 MINUTES- **COOKING TIME:** 15 MINUTES- **SERVINGS:** 4

CALORIES: 117, **CARBOHYDRATES:** 3g, **PROTEINS:** 4g, **FAT:** 9g

INGREDIENTS
1 1/2 cups steamed cauliflower
0.5oz butter
1/2 cup cream cheese
1/2 cup chilies
A pinch of pepper
A pinch of salt

DIRECTIONS
1) In a food processor, put all the ingredients
2) Grind well until the mixture is smooth
3) Using a teaspoon, divide the mixture into 6 equal servings
4) Air fry the mixture at 300F for 15 minutes
5) Serve freshly cooked

CINNAMON CUPCAKES

PREPARATION TIME: 15 MINUTES- **COOKING TIME:** 20 MINUTES- **SERVINGS:** 4

CALORIES: 150, **CARBOHYDRATES:** 5g, **PROTEINS:** 4g, **FAT:** 3g

INGREDIENTS
- ½ tablespoon of baking powder
- 1 teaspoon vanilla extract
- 1/2 cup almond flour
- 2 teaspoons cinnamon
- 0.5oz butter
- 4 tablespoons maple syrup
- 4 eggs
- Half an apple

DIRECTIONS
1) In a saucepan, heat the butter
2) Add the apple, eggs, maple syrup, and vanilla extract
3) Stir well
4) Let stand for 10 minutes
5) Add the flour, cinnamon, and baking powder
6) Mix well
7) Pour the mixture into the cupcake molds
8) Bake in the air fryer at 350F for 20 minutes
9) Let the cupcakes cool
10) Serve them at room temperature

CLASSIC FRANKFURTERS

PREPARATION TIME: 5 MINUTES- **COOKING TIME:** 10 MINUTES- **SERVINGS:** 4

CALORIES: 77, **CARBOHYDRATES:** 1g, **PROTEINS:** 8g, **FAT:** 5g

INGREDIENTS
- 10 ready-made Frankfurters
- Mayonnaise to taste

DIRECTIONS
1) Put the mayonnaise in each Frankfurter with the help of a pastry bag
2) Bake the Frankfurters in the air fryer at 350F for 10 minutes, turning them halfway through
3) Serve them freshly cooked

COCONUT AND VANILLA TREATS

PREPARATION TIME: 10 MINUTES- **COOKING TIME:** 12 MINUTES- **SERVINGS:** 4

CALORIES: 107, **CARBOHYDRATES:** 7g, **PROTEINS:** 5g, **FAT:** 3g

INGREDIENTS
- 1 cup almond flour
- 2 eggs
- 2 cups flaked coconut
- 1/4 cup milk

DIRECTIONS
1) Mix all the ingredients in a bowl, until smooth
2) Move the mixture to a baking pan
3) Bake in the air fryer at 350F for 12 minutes

CUCUMBER AND MOZZARELLA WRAP

PREPARATION TIME: 10 MINUTES - **COOKING TIME:** 5 MINUTES - **SERVINGS:** 4

CALORIES: 143, **CARBOHYDRATES:** 7g, **PROTEINS:** 8g. **FAT:** 8g

INGREDIENTS
1 cucumber
1 tablespoon water
1 mozzarella cheese
1 egg
2 ready-made tortilla wraps
0.5oz butter
A pinch of salt

DIRECTIONS
1) Beat the egg in a bowl
2) Add the mozzarella cheese, diced cucumber, water, and butter
3) Keep stirring to make a smooth mixture
4) Preheat the air fryer to 350F
5) Bake it for 5 minutes, until you get a nice golden crust
6) In a frying pan, heat the wraps
7) Fill each wrap with a generous amount of topping
8) Serve freshly cooked

GREEK-STYLE EGGS

PREPARATION TIME: 15 MINUTES - **COOKING TIME:** 10 MINUTES - **SERVINGS:** 4

CALORIES: 32, **CARBOHYDRATES:** 7g, **PROTEINS:** 1g, **FAT:** 1g

INGREDIENTS
1 tablespoon Greek yogurt
2 tablespoons pitted olives
3 eggs
A pinch of basil
A pinch of chopped chives
A pinch of pepper
A pinch of salt

DIRECTIONS
1) In the air fryer, Bake the eggs without opening them at 250F for 10 minutes
2) Move the eggs to a pan of cold water
3) Peel the eggs under running water
4) Cut the eggs in half, separating the white from the yolk
5) Mash the yolk together with the other ingredients, forming a kind of dough
6) Put the yolk back in its place
7) Serve the eggs freshly cooked

HEALTHY FRIES

PREPARATION TIME: 5 MINUTES- **COOKING TIME:** 20 MINUTES- **SERVINGS:** 4

CALORIES: 85, **CARBOHYDRATES:** 2g, **PROTEINS:** 5g, **FAT:** 6g

INGREDIENTS	DIRECTIONS
2 tablespoons Parmesan cheese 3 potatoes cut into the typical shape of French fries Salt to taste One tablespoon of olive oil A pinch of parsley	1) Mix potatoes together with Parmesan cheese, parsley, olive oil, and salt 2) Air fry at 350F for 20 minutes, stirring often 3) Serve them with a drizzle of mayonnaise

HERB CRAB CAKE

PREPARATION TIME: 20 MINUTES- **COOKING TIME:** 10 MINUTES- **SERVINGS:** 4

CALORIES: 107, **CARBOHYDRATES:** 2g, **PROTEINS:** 9g, **FAT:** 6g

INGREDIENTS	DIRECTIONS
1 teaspoon chili powder 1 egg 0.5oz butter 0.5oz crab meat 0.5oz almond flour A pinch of pepper A pinch of salt	1) Cut the crab meat into small pieces and place them in a bowl 2) Season the crabmeat with salt, pepper, and chili powder 3) Stir gently with a ladle 4) Add the egg and flour 5) Continue stirring until the mixture is smooth 6) In a small frying pan, melt the butter 7) Incorporate the butter into the mixture 8) Pour the mixture into the air fryer 9) Bake at 350F for 10 minutes, turning halfway through 10) Serve at room temperature

LEMON PIE

PREPARATION TIME: 100 MINUTES- **COOKING TIME:** 20 MINUTES- **SERVINGS:** 4

CALORIES: 82, CARBOHYDRATES: 2g, PROTEINS: 3g, FAT: 4g

INGREDIENTS
For the base:
- 2 drops of liquid stevia
- 3 tablespoons cold water
- 1/2 cup almond flour
- 1/2 cup butter
- A pinch of salt

For the filling:
- 1 teaspoon lemon juice
- 2 eggs
- 2 drops of liquid liquid stevia
- 1/2 cup butter
- The zest of two lemons

DIRECTIONS
1) In a bowl, mix the flour with the salt, and two tablespoons of liquid stevia
2) Combine the butter and water
3) Knead with your hands until smooth
4) Cover the dough and put it in the refrigerator for 60 minutes
5) Roll out the dough in a baking pan
6) Put it back in the refrigerator for another 20 minutes
7) In a bowl, combine the rest of the liquid stevia with the eggs, lemon juice, and lemon zest
8) Stir vigorously
9) Spread the resulting cream over the cake base
10) Bake at 350F for 20 minutes
11) Serve it freshly cooked

LENTILS AND DATES BROWNIES

PREPARATION TIME: 15 MINUTES- **COOKING TIME:** 15 MINUTES- **SERVINGS:** 4

CALORIES: 122, CARBOHYDRATES: 3g, PROTEINS: 4g, FAT: 4g

INGREDIENTS
- 1 peeled banana
- 1 tablespoon honey
- 12 dates
- 2 tablespoons cocoa powder
- 2 cups lentils
- 4 tablespoons peanut butter
- 2 tablespoons of baking powder

DIRECTIONS
1) Using a food processor, chop together the lentils with the peanut butter, banana, honey, cocoa, and baking powder
2) Add the dates, continuing to blend the mixture
3) Pour the mixture into a baking dish, distributing it evenly
4) Bake in the air fryer at 350F for 15 minutes
5) Serve freshly cooked

MELTED CHEESE CUPS

PREPARATION TIME: 10 MINUTES- **COOKING TIME** 12 MINUTES- **SERVINGS: 4**

CALORIES: 153, **CARBOHYDRATES**: 3g, **PROTEINS**: 5g, **FAT**: 3g

INGREDIENTS
- 3/4 cup cheese
- 2 eggs
- 1/2 cup bacon
- A pinch of paprika
- A pinch of pepper
- A pinch of salt

DIRECTIONS
1) Slice the bacon and sprinkle with salt, pepper, and paprika
2) Melt the butter in the bottom of the cups
3) Crack the eggs open, dividing them evenly among the cups
4) Add the cheese and bacon
5) Cook the cups in the air fryer at 350F for 12 minutes
6) Let the cups cool and serve at room temperature

MEXICAN-STYLE CHEESE STICKS

PREPARATION TIME: 10 MINUTES- **COOKING TIME**: 10 MINUTES- **SERVINGS: 4**

CALORIES: 169, **CARBOHYDRATES**: 3g, **PROTEINS**: 6g, **FAT**: 3g

INGREDIENTS
- 1 pinch of cumin
- 1 yolk
- 1 cup almond flour
- 2 cups cheese of your choice
- 1/2 cup Parmesan cheese
- A pinch of garlic powder

DIRECTIONS
1) Combine all the ingredients except the Parmesan cheese in a bowl
2) Mix until smooth
3) Divide the mixture into rectangles, resembling the shape of potato chips
4) Bake them at 350F for 10 minutes, turning them halfway through cooking
5) Let them cool before serving them with Parmesan cheese

MOZZARELLA CHEESE CUBES AND PAPRIKA

PREPARATION TIME: 10 MINUTES- **COOKING TIME**: 10 MINUTES- **SERVINGS: 4**

CALORIES: 162, **CARBOHYDRATES**: 1g, **PROTEINS**: 12g, **FAT**: 8g

INGREDIENTS
- 2 mozzarellas
- 1 3/4 cups of bacon
- Paprika to taste
- Pepper to taste

DIRECTIONS
1) Sprinkle the bacon with pepper and paprika
2) Cut the mozzarella into cubes
3) Wrap the mozzarella cubes in the bacon
4) Bake in the air fryer at 350F for 10 minutes
5) Serve the cubes freshly cooked

PUERTO RICAN-STYLE BANANA

PREPARATION TIME: 10 MINUTES- **COOKING TIME:** 10 MINUTES- **SERVINGS: 4**

CALORIES: 153, **CARBOHYDRATES:** 8g, **PROTEINS:** 5g, **FAT:** 4g

INGREDIENTS	DIRECTIONS
1 ripe banana 1 tablespoon sunflower seed oil A pinch of nutmeg A pinch of salt	1) Cut the banana in half lengthwise 2) Dip both sides in oil 3) Sprinkle both sides with nutmeg and salt 4) Bake the banana at 400F for 10 minutes, turning it every 2 minutes 5) Let the banana cool 6) Serve it at room temperature

ROASTED NUT MIX

PREPARATION TIME: 5 MINUTES- **COOKING TIME:** 8 MINUTES- **SERVINGS: 4**

CALORIES: 130, **CARBOHYDRATES:** 3g, **PROTEINS:** 9g, **FAT:** 4g

INGREDIENTS	DIRECTIONS
1 tablespoon olive oil 1/2 cup cashews 1/2 cup hazelnuts 1/2 cup macadamia nuts 1/2 cup pecans A pinch of salt	1) Bake the walnuts in the air fryer at 400F for 8 minutes, turning them halfway through 2) Drizzle the walnuts with olive oil and salt 3) Bake them for another minute 4) Let the nut mix cool 5) Serve it at room temperature

SEAWEED CHIPS

PREPARATION TIME: 5 MINUTES- **COOKING TIME:** 5 MINUTES- **SERVINGS: 4**

CALORIES: 4, **CARBOHYDRATES:** 1g, **PROTEINS:** 8g, **FAT:** 1g

INGREDIENTS	DIRECTIONS
1 teaspoon nutritional yeast 2 tablespoons water 3 sheets of nori seaweed	1) Cut the seaweed sheets as desired 2) Place them in the air fryer 3) Add the water and nutritional yeast 4) Bake at 350F for 5 minutes 5) Serve freshly cooked

SESAME-SEASONED BROCCOLI

PREPARATION TIME: 10 MINUTES- **COOKING TIME:** 10 MINUTES- **SERVINGS:** 4

CALORIES: 180, **CARBOHYDRATES:** 4g, **PROTEINS:** 5g, **FAT:** 13g

INGREDIENTS
- 1 tablespoon olive oil
- 2 tablespoons rice vinegar
- 2 tablespoons of sesame oil
- 2 1/2 cups of broccoli
- A pinch of salt

DIRECTIONS
1) Preheat the air fryer to 400F
2) In a bowl, place the broccoli, olive oil, and salt
3) Stir vigorously
4) Bake the broccoli in the air fryer for 10 minutes, turning it halfway through cooking
5) Mix the vinegar and sesame oil in a bowl
6) Transfer the broccoli to the bowl
7) Stir until the sauce has soaked them thoroughly
8) Serve the broccoli at room temperature

SOFT CAKE

PREPARATION TIME: 25 MINUTES- **COOKING TIME:** 20 MINUTES- **SERVINGS:** 4

CALORIES: 146, **CARBOHYDRATES:** 6g, **PROTEINS:** 2g, **FAT:** 3g

INGREDIENTS
- 3 tablespoons of baking powder
- 4 cups of milk
- 2 teaspoons vanilla extract
- 2 cups olive oil
- 2 drops of liquid stevia
- 2 cups water
- 1/2 cup lemon juice
- 3 cups almond flour

DIRECTIONS
1) In one bowl, mix the flour, cornstarch, baking powder, and liquid stevia
2) In a second bowl, mix the oil with the milk, water, vanilla, and lemon juice
3) Combine the two compounds
4) Bake in the air fryer at 350F for 20 minutes
5) Let it cool
6) Serve the cake at room temperature

SPICY BACON BITES

PREPARATION TIME: 15 MINUTES- **COOKING TIME:** 11 MINUTES- **SERVINGS: 4**

CALORIES: 153, **CARBOHYDRATES:** 8g, **PROTEINS:** 5g, **FAT:** 4g

INGREDIENTS
1 tablespoon olive oil
2 cups jalapeno peppers
1 1/4 cup sliced bacon
One teaspoon paprika
A pinch of salt

DIRECTIONS
1) Wash the chilies well
2) Mix the salt, paprika, and olive oil
3) Dip the chiles in the freshly prepared sauce
4) Roll each jalapeno in a slice of bacon
5) Air fry at 350F for 11 minutes or until bacon is crispy
6) Wipe off excess oil on the chiles with a paper towel
7) Serve them freshly cooked

STRAWBERRY SWEETS

PREPARATION TIME: 25 MINUTES- **COOKING TIME:** 45 MINUTES- **SERVINGS: 4**

CALORIES: 164, **CARBOHYDRATES:** 5g, **PROTEINS:** 2g, **FAT:** 2g

INGREDIENTS
3 tablespoons of baking powder
1 teaspoon of rum
1 egg
3 cups almond flour
2 drops of liquid liquid stevia
1/2 cup strawberries
1/2 cup butter
The peel of one lemon

DIRECTIONS
1) In a bowl, mix the flour with the liquid stevia and baking powder
2) In another bowl, beat the eggs
3) Combine the eggs with the flour
4) Divide the dough into 6 equal parts
5) Bake in the air fryer at 350F for 45 minutes
6) In a bowl, mix the strawberries with the rum and lemon zest
7) Place the freshly prepared strawberries on each cupcake
8) Serve the treats at room temperature

TACO CHIPS

PREPARATION TIME: 5 MINUTES- COOKING TIME: 2 MINUTES- SERVINGS: 4

CALORIES: 50, CARBOHYDRATES: 3g, PROTEINS: 7g, FAT: 1g

INGREDIENTS
- 2 tacos
- Salt to taste
- One tablespoon of olive oil

DIRECTIONS

1) Cut the tacos into wedges
2) Sprinkle the tacos with oil and salt
3) Bake them in the air fryer at 350F for 2 minutes
4) Serve them as an appetizer

TANGERINE PUDDING

PREPARATION TIME: 5 MINUTES- COOKING TIME: 40 MINUTES- SERVINGS: 4

CALORIES: 62, CARBOHYDRATES: 3g, PROTEINS: 6g, FAT: 3g

INGREDIENTS
- 1 peeled tangerine
- 1/2 cup almond flour
- 2 drops of liquid liquid stevia
- 2 medium eggs
- 0.5oz butter

DIRECTIONS

1) In a baking dish combine all the ingredients except the honey
2) Bake in the air fryer at 350F for 40 minutes
3) Serve freshly cooked using honey as topping

ZUCCHINI CHIPS

PREPARATION TIME: 5 MINUTES-COOKING TIME: 35 MINUTES- SERVINGS: 4

CALORIES: 16, CARBOHYDRATES: 3g, PROTEINS: 2g, FAT: 2g

INGREDIENTS
- 1 teaspoon salt
- 3 cut zucchini

DIRECTIONS

1) Put the zucchini in the air fryer and sprinkle them with salt
2) Bake them at 350F for 35 minutes, turning them every 5 minutes
3) Serve them freshly cooked

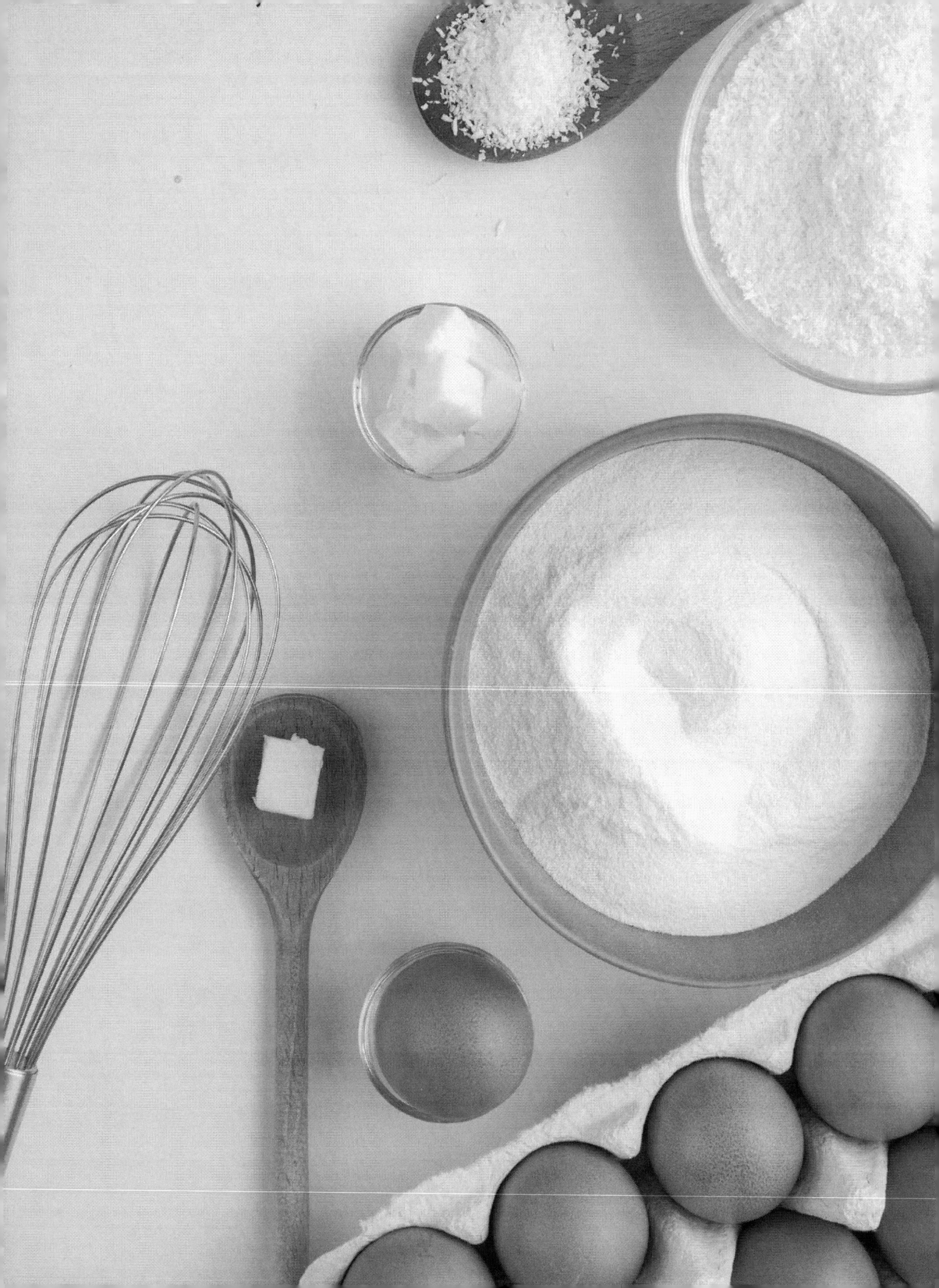

DESSERTS

The art of baking is more than cooking: it is an act of love.

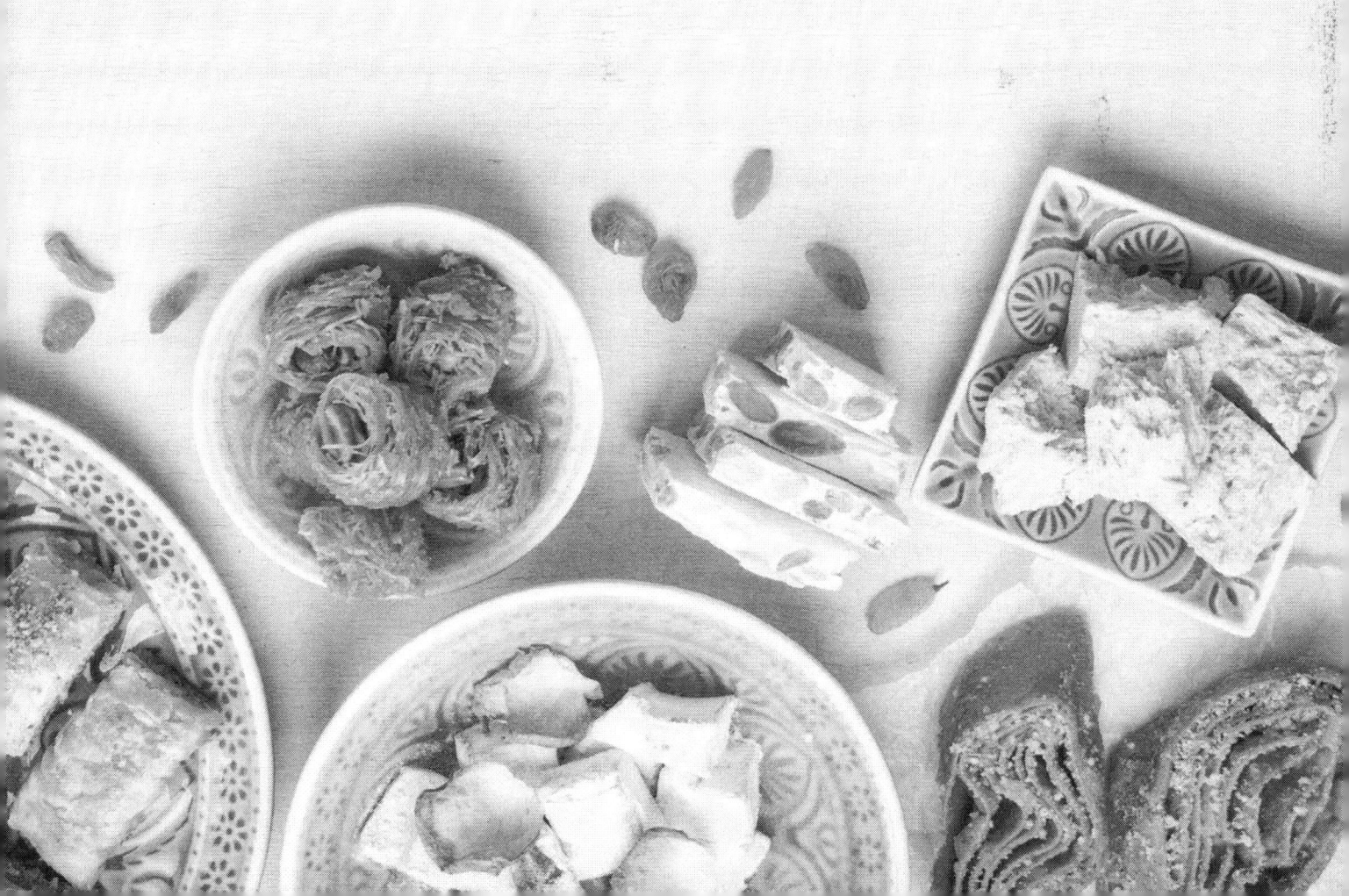

AIR FRIED BISCUITS

PREPARATION TIME: 15 MINUTES- **COOKING TIME:** 10 MINUTES- **SERVINGS:** 4

CALORIES: 17, **CARBOHYDRATES:** 2g, **PROTEINS:** 5g, **FAT:** 8g

INGREDIENTS
2 marshmallows
4 of your favorite cookies
4 pieces of chocolate

DIRECTIONS
1) Break the cookies in half to create 8 pieces
2) Cut the marshmallows in half with a pair of scissors
3) Place the marshmallow pieces on 4 of the 8 cookie pieces
4) Bake in the air fryer at 380F for 10 minutes or until golden brown
5) Add the chocolate
6) Close the cookies with the other halves, like small sandwiches
7) Serve them freshly cooked

ALMOND COOKIES

PREPARATION TIME: 15 MINUTES- **COOKING TIME:** 15 MINUTES- **SERVINGS:** 4

CALORIES: 116, **CARBOHYDRATES:** 3g, **PROTEINS:** 13g, **FAT:** 4g

INGREDIENTS
1 teaspoon almond extract
1 cup butter
1 cup almonds
2 cups almond flour
A pinch of salt
2 drops of liquid liquid stevia

DIRECTIONS
1) In a bowl, mix the liquid stevia with the almond extract
2) Add the flour
3) Continue stirring until a malleable dough forms
4) Divide the dough according to the number of cookies you want to make
5) Put the cookies in the air fryer
6) Bake in the air fryer at 350F for 15 minutes, until the edges begin to turn golden brown
7) Serve them freshly cooked

ALMONDS AND PEANUT BUTTER BALLS

PREPARATION TIME: 15 MINUTES- **COOKING TIME:** 10 MINUTES- **SERVINGS: 4**

CALORIES: 124, **CARBOHYDRATES:** 3g, **PROTEINS:** 11g, **FAT:** 3g

INGREDIENTS
- 1 teaspoon vanilla extract
- 1 egg
- 2 cups peanut butter
- 1/2 cup unsweetened flaked coconut
- 1/2 cup chocolate chips

DIRECTIONS
1) In a bowl, mix all the ingredients
2) Helping yourself with your hands, create small spheres
3) Bake the spheres in the air fryer at 350F for 10 minutes
4) Let the spheres cool completely
5) Store them in the refrigerator and consume them within 4 days

APPLE AND RAISIN PASTRIES

PREPARATION TIME: 10 MINUTES- **COOKING TIME:** 25 MINUTES- **SERVINGS: 4**

CALORIES: 120, **CARBOHYDRATES:** 7g, **PROTEINS:** 5g, **FAT:** 4g

INGREDIENTS
- 2 drops of liquid liquid stevia
- 2 tablespoons melted butter
- 2 apples
- 2 rolls of puff pastry

DIRECTIONS
1) Preheat the air fryer to 350F
2) Peel the apples and cut them into small pieces
3) In a bowl, combine the apples and the liquid stevia
4) Mix well
5) Put the filling on one roll of puff pastry
6) Use the second roll to close the pastry
7) Using a knife, divide the pastry into many small servings
8) Spread melted butter on the surface of the pastries
9) Bake them for 25 minutes
10) Serve them freshly cooked

APPLE CHIPS

PREPARATION TIME: 10 MINUTES- COOKING TIME: 8 MINUTES- SERVINGS: 4

CALORIES: 108, CARBOHYDRATES: 5g, PROTEINS: 7g, FAT: 2g

INGREDIENTS
2 drops of liquid liquid stevia
1 apple
Half a teaspoon of cinnamon
A pinch of salt

DIRECTIONS
1) Cut up the apples
2) Sprinkle them with cinnamon, liquid stevia, and salt
3) Turn them over and do the same on the other side
4) Air fry the apples at 350F for 8 minutes, turning them halfway through
5) Serve them freshly cooked

APPLE CINNAMON PIE

PREPARATION TIME: 25 MINUTES- COOKING TIME: 45 MINUTES- SERVINGS: 4

CALORIES: 55, CARBOHYDRATES: 9g, PROTEINS: 3g, FAT: 0g

INGREDIENTS
Crust:
1 roll of puff pastry
1 egg
2 teaspoons cinnamon
0.5oz butter
Cake:
1 3/4 cups butter
2 cups almond flour
2 drops of liquid liquid stevia
7 apples
Filling:
2 drops of liquid liquid stevia
2 tablespoons milk
A pinch of cinnamon

DIRECTIONS
1) Preheat the air fryer to 350F
2) Unroll the puff pastry
3) Spread it with butter
4) Sprinkle cinnamon on top
5) Sprinkle the puff pastry with the egg
6) Add the sliced apples
7) Add the flour, liquid stevia, and butter
8) Bake in the air fryer for 45 minutes
9) In a bowl, mix the ingredients for the filling until creamy
10) Finish the cake by adding milk, liquid stevia, and cinnamon filling
11) Serve the cake freshly cooked

APPLE PASTRIES

PREPARATION TIME: 10 MINUTES- **COOKING TIME:** 8 MINUTES- **SERVINGS: 4**

CALORIES: 78, **CARBOHYDRATES:** 7g, **PROTEINS:** 5g, **FAT:** 2g

INGREDIENTS
1 roll of puff pastry
5 apples

DIRECTIONS
1) Cut the apples into slices
2) Unroll the puff pastry in a baking dish
3) Arrange the apples on the puff pastry
4) Close the puff pastry, forming the shape of a pastry
5) Bake the pie in the air fryer at 350F for 8 minutes or until the pastry is golden brown
6) Serve freshly cooked

APPLE ROLLS

PREPARATION TIME: 15 MINUTES- **COOKING TIME:** 25 MINUTES- **SERVINGS: 4**

CALORIES: 47, **CARBOHYDRATES:** 2g, **PROTEINS:** 6g, **FAT:** 1g

INGREDIENTS
1 roll of puff pastry
1 egg
2 sliced apples
2 drops of liquid liquid stevia

DIRECTIONS
1) Preheat the air fryer to 350F
2) Unroll the puff pastry
3) Arrange the apples evenly on the pastry
4) Roll up the puff pastry, being careful not to let the apples come out
5) With a brush, spread egg on the surface of the pastry
6) Add the liquid stevia
7) Bake for 25 minutes
8) Serve the roll freshly cooked

APPLE-FLAVORED BITES

PREPARATION TIME: 15 MINUTES- **COOKING TIME:** 15 MINUTES- **SERVINGS:** 4

CALORIES: 49.7, **CARBOHYDRATES:** 7g, **PROTEINS:** 1g, **FAT:** 3g

INGREDIENTS
1 apple
2 rolls of puff pastry
0.5oz butter
0.5oz finely chopped hazelnuts
3 teaspoons cinnamon

DIRECTIONS
1) Preheat the air fryer to 350F
2) Unroll the puff pastry on a baking sheet
3) In a small saucepan, melt the butter
4) Spread the butter on the puff pastry
5) Sprinkle the puff pastry with the cinnamon and liquid stevia
6) Add the hazelnuts and apples
7) Using the second roll of puff pastry, cover the first roll, forming a casket
8) Bake for 15 minutes
9) Cut the casket into many smaller pieces
10) Serve the apple bites freshly cooked

BUTTER AND STEVIA PIE

PREPARATION TIME: 5 MINUTES- **COOKING TIME:** 35 MINUTES- **SERVINGS:** 4

CALORIES: 95, **CARBOHYDRATES:** 5g, **PROTEINS:** 4g, **FAT:** 3g

INGREDIENTS
1 tablespoon of baking powder
1 teaspoon cinnamon
2 drops of liquid liquid stevia
3 eggs
1 1/4 cup butter
1 1/4 cup almond flour
0.5oz milk

DIRECTIONS
1) Preheat to 350F
2) Combine all the ingredients in a bowl
3) Mix well
4) Bake for 35 minutes in the air fryer
5) Let the cake cool
6) Serve it at room temperature

CAKE BITES

PREPARATION TIME: 15 MINUTES- **COOKING TIME:** 7 MINUTES- **SERVINGS:** 4

CALORIES: 150, **CARBOHYDRATES:** 4g, **PROTEINS:** 13g, **FAT:** 3g

INGREDIENTS
2 cups almond flour
2 tablespoons baking powder
2 cups Greek yogurt
2 drops of liquid liquid stevia

DIRECTIONS
1) In a bowl, mix yogurt and flour until a smooth dough is obtained
2) Add the baking powder and the stevia
3) Cut the dough into 32 squares
4) Bake them in the air fryer at 350F for 4 minutes
5) Turn them over and bake them for another 3 minutes
6) Serve them freshly cooked

CARAMEL AND COCONUT CREAM

PREPARATION TIME: 10 MINUTES- **COOKING TIME:** 15 MINUTES- **SERVINGS: 4**

CALORIES: 31, **CARBOHYDRATES:** 2g, **PROTEINS:** 4g, **FAT:** 0g

INGREDIENTS
- 1 teaspoon cinnamon
- 2 drops of liquid liquid stevia
- 1 cup of sour cream
- 3 tablespoons caramel syrup
- 1/2 cup coconut cream

DIRECTIONS
1) In a bowl, mix the sour cream with the caramel syrup
2) Add the other ingredients
3) Mix well
4) Bake in the air fryer at 350F for 15 minutes
5) Serve the cream freshly cooked

CHERRY PIE

PREPARATION TIME: 10 MINUTES- **COOKING TIME:** 15 MINUTES- **SERVINGS: 4**

CALORIES: 100, **CARBOHYDRATES:** 11g, **PROTEINS:** 7g, **FAT:** 4g

INGREDIENTS
- 1 tablespoon milk
- 1 yolk
- 1 jar of cherry jam
- 2 rolls of puff pastry
- Vanilla ice cream as much as needed

DIRECTIONS
1) Heat the air fryer to 350F
2) Unroll the puff pastry in a baking dish
3) Poke holes in the pastry with a fork
4) Fill the center with cherry jam
5) Close the pie with the second roll of puff pastry
6) Trim off excess pastry
7) Bake in the air fryer for 15 minutes
8) Serve with a scoop of vanilla ice cream

CHOCOLATE AND PEANUT BUTTER COOKIES

PREPARATION TIME: 25 MINUTES- **COOKING TIME:** 10 MINUTES- **SERVINGS: 4**

CALORIES: 72, CARBOHYDRATES: 5g, PROTEINS: 6g, FAT: 2g

INGREDIENTS
- 2 tablespoons of baking powder
- 1 tablespoon vanilla extract
- 1 egg
- 1 cup peanut butter
- 2 drops of liquid liquid stevia
- 2 cups almond flour
- 1/2 cup peanuts
- 1/2 cup cocoa powder
- A pinch of salt

DIRECTIONS
1) Preheat the air fryer to 320F
2) In a small saucepan, melt the butter
3) Mix the butter, peanut butter, and liquid stevia in a bowl
4) Add the eggs and vanilla
5) Continue stirring until the mixture is smooth
6) Add the salt, baking powder, cocoa powder, and flour
7) Continue mixing until a dough is created
8) Roll out the dough with a rolling pin
9) Cut out cookies in the shape you prefer
10) Bake the cookies for 10 minutes
11) Let them cool for at least 5 minutes

CHOCOLATE CUPCAKE WITH CHOCOLATE CREAM

PREPARATION TIME: 10 MINUTES- **COOKING TIME:** 20 MINUTES- **SERVINGS: 4**

CALORIES: 104, CARBOHYDRATES: 3g, PROTEINS: 12g, FAT: 5g

INGREDIENTS
- 3/4 cup dark chocolate pieces
- 1 cup butter
- 2 drops of liquid stevia
- 2 eggs
- 1/2 cup almond flour
- ½ tablespoon of baking powder

DIRECTIONS
1) Preheat the air fryer to 350F
2) In a small saucepan, melt the butter and chocolate
3) Add the liquid stevia and eggs, continuing to stir
4) Add the other ingredients
5) Pour into the molds
6) Put the molds in the air fryer
7) Bake for 10 minutes
8) Flip the molds onto a plate and serve the cupcakes freshly cooked

CHOCOLATE MUG CAKE

PREPARATION TIME: 10 MINUTES- **COOKING TIME:** 13 MINUTES- **SERVINGS: 4**

CALORIES: 129, **CARBOHYDRATES:** 8g, **PROTEINS:** 5g, **FAT:** 4g

INGREDIENTS
- 1 tablespoon of cocoa powder
- 3 tablespoons milk
- 2 drops of liquid stevia
- 1/2 cup almond flour
- ½ tablespoon of baking powder

DIRECTIONS
1) In a bowl, combine all the ingredients
2) Mix them well together
3) Bake in the air fryer at 190F for 13 minutes
4) Serve at room temperature

CHOCOLATE SUFFLÈ

PREPARATION TIME: 10 MINUTES- **COOKING TIME:** 14 MINUTES- **SERVINGS: 4**

CALORIES: 138, **CARBOHYDRATES:** 4g, **PROTEINS:** 9g, **FAT:** 3g

INGREDIENTS
- 1 cup milk chocolate
- 2 tablespoons almond flour
- 2 eggs
- 2 drops of liquid liquid stevia
- 1/4 cup seed oil
- A dash of vanilla extract

DIRECTIONS
1) Melt together the oil and chocolate
2) Beat the egg yolks
3) Add the vanilla and liquid stevia
4) Add the flour
5) Stir making sure there are no lumps
6) Preheat the air fryer to 330F
7) Whip the whites to stiff peaks
8) Combine the whites with the chocolate
9) Combine all parts
10) Bake for 14 minutes

CINNAMON PEAR CHIPS

PREPARATION TIME: 10 MINUTES- **COOKING TIME:** 25 MINUTES- **SERVINGS: 4**

CALORIES: 98, **CARBOHYDRATES:** 1g, **PROTEINS:** 6g, **FAT:** 1g

INGREDIENTS
- 1 tablespoon cinnamon
- 1 cup butter
- 1 cup almond flour
- 2 pears cut into cubes
- 2 drops of liquid stevia

DIRECTIONS
1) Mix the flour and butter in a bowl
2) Add cinnamon and liquid stevia
3) Put the pears in the air fryer
4) Pour the mixture of flour, butter, cinnamon, and liquid stevia over the pears
5) Bake at 350F for 25 minutes
6) Serve the chips freshly cooked

COCONUT AND HONEY APRICOTS

PREPARATION TIME: 10 MINUTES- **COOKING TIME:** 16 MINUTES- **SERVINGS:** 4

CALORIES: 150, **CARBOHYDRATES:** 1g, **PROTEINS:** 8g, **FAT:** 7g

INGREDIENTS
1 teaspoon cinnamon
1 tablespoon flaked coconut
1 tablespoon honey
3/4 cup mascarpone cheese
8 apricots cut in half

DIRECTIONS
1) Sprinkle the apricots with coconut flakes
2) Bake in the air fryer at 350F for 16 minutes
3) Add the mascarpone, honey, and cinnamon
4) Serve them freshly cooked

CURRANT AND CHOCOLATE CUPCAKES

PREPARATION TIME: 15 MINUTES- **COOKING TIME:** 15 MINUTES- **SERVINGS:** 4

CALORIES: 145, **CARBOHYDRATES:** 6g, **PROTEINS:** 16g, **FAT:** 4g

INGREDIENTS
For the cupcakes:
3/4 cup currants
1 cup butter
1/2 cup almond flour
½ tablespoon of baking powder
2 drops of liquid stevia
1/2 cup cocoa powder
A pinch of salt
For the icing:
1 teaspoon vanilla extract
1 cup butter
1 cup of chocolate chips

DIRECTIONS
1) Preheat the air fryer to 350F
2) In a bowl, mix all the ingredients for the cupcakes
3) Place the molds in the air fryer
4) Fill the molds with the batter
5) Bake the cupcakes at 350F for 15 minutes
6) Using a food processor, mix all the ingredients for the frosting
7) Using a piping bag, decorate the cupcakes with the frosting
8) Serve the cupcakes at room temperature

DANISH CINNAMON ROLLS

PREPARATION TIME: 5 MINUTES- **COOKING TIME:** 10 MINUTES- **SERVINGS:** 4

CALORIES: 122, **CARBOHYDRATES:** 2g, **PROTEINS:** 6g, **FAT:** 3g

INGREDIENTS
1 teaspoon cinnamon
1 tablespoon seed oil
2 rolls of puff pastry
2 drops of liquid stevia

DIRECTIONS
1) Cut the puff pastry into rectangles
2) In a bowl, mix the other ingredients
3) Fill each rectangle with the resulting sauce
4) Close each puff pastry rectangle carefully
5) Bake the rolls in the air fryer at 300F for 10 minutes, turning them halfway through
6) Serve them freshly cooked

DEEP-FRIED BANANAS WITH CHOCOLATE SAUCE

PREPARATION TIME: 10 MINUTES- **COOKING TIME:** 7 MINUTES- **SERVINGS: 4**

CALORIES: 103, **CARBOHYDRATES:** 3g, **PROTEINS:** 8g, **FAT:** 3g

INGREDIENTS
- 1 tablespoon of seed oil
- 1 egg
- 3 bananas cut lengthwise
- 1/2 cup cornstarch
- 1/2 cup of breadcrumbs
- Chocolate spread of your choice

DIRECTIONS
1) In one bowl, beat the egg
2) Put the cornstarch in a second bow
3) In a third bowl, put the breadcrumbs
4) Mash the bananas in the cornstarcH
5) Pass the bananas into the egg
6) Pass the bananas into the breadcrumbs
7) Air fry the bananas at 350F for 5 minutes
8) Turn them over and cook them for another 2 minutes
9) Spread the chocolate cream on the bananas
10) Serve them freshly cooked

EASY BISCUITS

PREPARATION TIME: 10 MINUTES- **COOKING TIME:** 15 MINUTES- **SERVINGS: 4**

CALORIES: 82, **CARBOHYDRATES:** 3g, **PROTEINS:** 3g, **FAT:** 6g

INGREDIENTS
- 1 teaspoon vanilla extract
- 1 cup butter
- 2 drops of liquid stevia
- 2 cups flour
- A pinch of salt

DIRECTIONS
1) Preheat the air fryer to 300F
2) In a bowl, mix butter and liquid stevia until soft and smooth
3) Incorporate the vanilla and flour
4) Divide the dough into equal parts
5) Bake the cookies for 15 minutes
6) Let them cool for 10 minutes
7) Serve them at room temperature

FRIED CINNAMON BANANAS

PREPARATION TIME: 5 MINUTES- **COOKING TIME:** 13 MINUTES- **SERVINGS:** 4

CALORIES 163, CARBOHYDRATES: 2g, PROTEINS: 3g, FAT: 12g

INGREDIENTS
1 banana peeled and cut into rounds
1 tablespoon of seed oil
2 drops of liquid stevia
A pinch of cinnamon

DIRECTIONS
1) Preheat the air fryer to 400F
2) Mix all the ingredients
3) Air fry the banana rounds for about 13 minutes, turning them halfway through
4) Serve them freshly cooked

FRIED PLANTAINS

PREPARATION TIME: 10 MINUTES- **COOKING TIME:** 10 MINUTES- **SERVINGS:** 4

CALORIES: 100, CARBOHYDRATES: 11g, PROTEINS: 7g, FAT: 4g

INGREDIENTS
1 egg white
1/2 cup of breadcrumbs
3 tablespoons of oil
8 small bananas

DIRECTIONS
1) Preheat the air fryer to 350F
2) In a small pan, cook breadcrumbs with oil until golden brown
3) Coat the bananas with the egg white and breadcrumbs
4) Air fry the bananas for 10 minutes
5) Serve them at room temperature

HAZELNUT CAKE

PREPARATION TIME: 5 MINUTES- **COOKING TIME:** 10 MINUTES- **SERVINGS:** 4

CALORIES: 75, CARBOHYDRATES: 2g, PROTEINS: 1g, FAT: 6g

INGREDIENTS
1 tablespoon of baking powder
1 tablespoon of seed oil
1 cup almond flour
2 eggs
1/2 cup chopped hazelnuts

DIRECTIONS
1) In a bowl, mix all the ingredients until smooth
2) Bake in the air fryer at 350F for 10 minutes, turning the mixture halfway through
3) Serve the cake at room temperature

LEMON BUTTER COOKIES

PREPARATION TIME: 25 MINUTES- **COOKING TIME:** 15 MINUTES- **SERVINGS: 4**

CALORIES: 89, **CARBOHYDRATES:** 3g, **PROTEINS:** 3g, **FAT:** 9g

INGREDIENTS
- 1 teaspoon vanilla extract
- 1 cup butter
- 2 drops of liquid stevia
- 2 cups almond flour
- The zest of one lemon
- A pinch of salt

DIRECTIONS
1) Preheat the air fryer to 350F
2) In a bowl, mix the butter with the liquid stevia until soft and smooth
3) Add the vanilla extract and lemon zest
4) Add the flour as well
5) Continue mixing until a malleable dough forms
6) Divide the dough into many small cookies
7) Bake for 15 minutes
8) Let the cookies cool for 10 minutes before serving

PEANUT BUTTER AND MARSHMALLOW CROISSANTS

PREPARATION TIME: 15 MINUTES- **COOKING TIME:** 5 MINUTES- **SERVINGS: 4**

CALORIES: 84, **CARBOHYDRATES:** 3g, **PROTEINS:** 5g, **FAT:** 2g

INGREDIENTS
- 1 pinch of salt
- 2 rolls of puff pastry
- 0.5oz melted butter
- 4 tablespoons peanut butter
- 4 teaspoons marshmallow cream

DIRECTIONS
1) Preheat the air fryer to 350F
2) On one roll of puff pastry, spread melted butter
3) Place the second roll on top of the first
4) Spread it too with melted butter
5) Cut the pastry into 4 squares
6) On each square, place a spoonful of marshmallow and peanut butter cream
7) Fold each square in half, forming a triangle
8) Make sure the filling is tightly enclosed in the dough
9) Bake in the air fryer at 350F for 5 minutes
10) Add a pinch of salt to give the sweet-savory effect
11) Serve the croissants freshly cooked

PINEAPPLE YOGURT STICKS

PREPARATION TIME: 10 MINUTES- **COOKING TIME:** 10 MINUTES- **SERVINGS:** 4

CALORIES: 100, **CARBOHYDRATES:** 4g, **PROTEINS:** 7g, **FAT:** 4g

INGREDIENTS
2 cups vanilla yogurt
Half a pineapple
A handful of fresh mint

DIRECTIONS
1) Preheat the air fryer to 350F
2) Cut the pineapple into pieces
3) Air fry the pineapple for 10 minutes
4) Chop the mint finely
5) Mix the mint with the yogurt
6) Serve the pineapple sticks with the yogurt and mint

RUM PANCAKES

PREPARATION TIME: 10 MINUTES- **COOKING TIME:** 10 MINUTES- **SERVINGS:** 4

CALORIES: 138, **CARBOHYDRATES:** 4g, **PROTEINS:** 5g, **FAT:** 1g

INGREDIENTS
1 mashed banana
1 tablespoon rum
2 drops of liquid stevia
1/2 cup almond flour
3/4 cup water
1/2 cup butter
A pinch of nutmeg

DIRECTIONS
1) In a bowl, mix all the ingredients
2) Pour the dough into the air fryer
3) Using your hands, divide the dough into about 10 parts
4) Bake in the air fryer at 350F for 10 minutes, turning the pancakes halfway through cooking
5) Serve the pancakes freshly cooked

STRAWBERRY SHORTCAKES

PREPARATION TIME: 25 MINUTES- **COOKING TIME:** 10 MINUTES- **SERVINGS: 4**

CALORIES: 118, **CARBOHYDRATES:** 9g, **PROTEINS:** 22g, **FAT:** 6g

INGREDIENTS
- 1 roll of puff pastry
- 2 drops of liquid stevia
- 1 cup strawberries
- The juice of one lemon

DIRECTIONS
1) Cut the strawberries
2) Mix them in a bowl with liquid stevia and lemon juice
3) Let the strawberries rest for 15 minutes
4) Cut the puff pastry into 12 small rectangles
5) Put about 2 teaspoons of strawberries in the center of 6 rectangles, leaving a half-inch border
6) Cover the 6 filled rectangles with the unstuffed ones
7) Bake in the air fryer at 350F for 10 minutes

VANILLA COOKIES

PREPARATION TIME: 10 MINUTES- **COOKING TIME:** 20 MINUTES- **SERVINGS: 4**

CALORIES: 134, **CARBOHYDRATES:** 4g, **PROTEINS:** 17g, **FAT:** 3g

INGREDIENTS
- 1 tablespoon sour cream
- 1 cup of melted butter
- 1/2 cup almond flour
- 2 teaspoons vanilla extract
- 2 beaten eggs
- 2 drops of liquid stevia

DIRECTIONS
1) In a bowl, mix all the ingredients
2) Scoop out 12 balls
3) Place them in the air fryer
4) Bake in the air fryer at 350F for 20 minutes
5) Serve the cookies at room temperature

VANILLA-CINNAMON COOKIES

PREPARATION TIME: 10 MINUTES- **COOKING TIME:** 15 MINUTES- **SERVINGS: 4**

CALORIES: 120, **CARBOHYDRATES:** 4g, **PROTEINS:** 13g, **FAT:** 5g

INGREDIENTS
- 1 teaspoon vanilla extract
- 1 egg
- 2 teaspoons grated ginger
- 1/2 cup almond flour
- 1/2 cup melted butter
- A pinch of cinnamon
- A pinch of nutmeg

DIRECTIONS
1) In a bowl, mix all the ingredients
2) Helping yourself with a spoon, form small balls of dough
3) Place them in the air fryer
4) Bake the balls at 350F for 15 minutes
5) Let the cookies cool
6) Serve them at room temperature

VANILLA MUG CAKE

PREPARATION TIME: 10 MINUTES - **COOKING TIME:** 20 MINUTES - **SERVINGS: 4**

CALORIES: 151, **CARBOHYDRATES:** 3g, **PROTEINS:** 5g, **FAT:** 2g

INGREDIENTS
1 teaspoon vanilla extract
1 teaspoon baking powder
2 tablespoons cocoa powder
2 tablespoons milk
2 tablespoons agave juice
2 teaspoons coconut oil

DIRECTIONS
1) Preheat the air fryer to 350F
2) In a bowl, mix all the ingredients until smooth
3) Put the resulting mixture into a bowl
4) Bake for about 20 minutes
5) Serve the mug cake freshly cooked

BONUS GUIDES

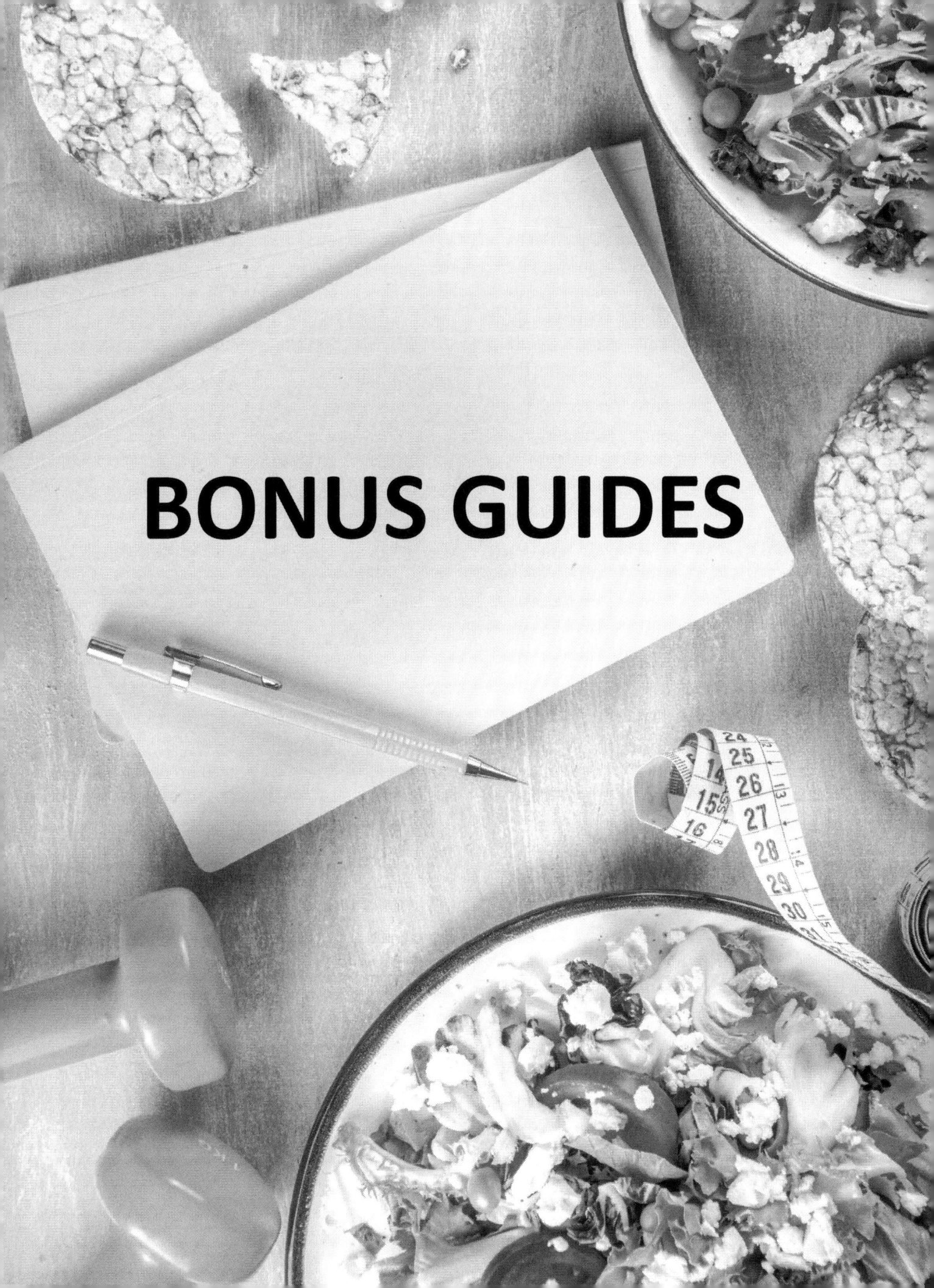

TIPS AND TRICKS TO PREVENT HAIR LOSS

After undergoing bariatric surgery, the body changes and has to get used to the new condition that affects the digestive system, and the way micronutrients are absorbed.

Hair loss is among the "side effects" of particular concern to those who have undergone bariatric surgery. Always synonymous with beauty and seduction, hair loss is experienced with considerable discomfort. Indeed, with bariatric surgery, the patient not only aims to improve his or her health but also subconsciously desires to rebuild a better appearance that can facilitate human relationships, love life, and social inclusion. However, in the following paragraphs, we will explain why this happens and why it should not raise strong concerns in the patient.

In the first six months following the operation, we may notice a thinning of the foliage due to an adaptation phase of the organism. This process, we make it clear now, is reversible and momentary. The situation improves as we expand the diet, which can be combined with bariatric supplements specially formulated to meet the nutritional needs of patients who have undergone malabsorptive or restrictive surgery.

Every day we lose hair; we notice this phenomenon when we comb our hair or shampoo. However, we are not alarmed because the hair that falls out is replaced by new hair.

This mechanism, after bariatric surgery, slows down. Hair loss then may correspond to the physiological loss that we observe daily. What changes is the speed of regrowth. What does this mean? The body, after bariatric surgery, must cope with significant change, and to do so efficiently, it slows down some functions, including hair regrowth.

Once the body adjusts to the new physiological condition, we see an upswing in hair regrowth. As often said, bariatric surgery limits food intake and nutrient absorption. In case of nutritional deficiencies, the attending physician might combine the diet with a supplement specifically for bariatric patients.

In detail, after bariatric surgery, we may see nutritional deficiencies involving nutrients such as Group B Vitamins, Vitamin A, Vitamin C, Vitamin E, Niacin, Iron, Magnesium, and Zinc. The latter contribute, in different ways, to hair bulb proliferation, growth mechanisms, and hair structure, as well as being involved in other physiological processes.

Taking a supplement formulated specifically for the bariatric surgery patient can help fill nutritional deficiencies, which cannot be resolved through diet, to restore the balance of vitamins and minerals, which are helpful for the body to preside over various physiological functions.

Another tip for preventing post-op hair loss is to drink plenty of water.

My advice is to drink at least 2 liters of water a day, although it may seem complicated because of the small size of the stomach. Keeping well hydrated, however, avoids complications such as hair loss, vision problems, and skin flaking.

Furthermore, achieving daily protein intake is also very important to prevent and slow down hair loss. In this case, it is essential to slavishly follow the instructions given by our nutritionist, no matter how much we feel like eating what is prescribed.

HOW TO OVERCOME STALLS

Most people who have undergone bariatric surgery have experienced what is known as a "plateau" or stall, that is, a phase of slowing or stalling weight loss, sometimes even regaining a few pounds. This mechanism, rather frustrating for those trying to get in shape, is a natural defense of the body that responds to the stimulus of slimming, perceiving it as a threat to its health and good functioning and opposing it. The body functions according to the principle of homeostasis, or the ability to keep itself balanced and functioning even when disrupted by external events by adapting to them. In the case of obesity, the body becomes accustomed to having a certain metabolic and hormonal value depending on the amount of fat. However, in the long term, a very high weight can have serious health complications, and the body becomes accustomed to it by perceiving it as healthy. If adipose is lost in large amounts, our body works by creating micro-strategies not to lose anymore until it has adapted to the new weight, for example, by lowering energy consumption.

This situation is not forever and especially not irreversible; we just need to understand what specifically caused the plateau and intervene appropriately, usually by creating a kind of a small shock to the metabolism that spurs it to react promptly.

For example, the most common cause of stalling is a rigidly low-calorie diet designed to lose many pounds (8-10) in a couple of months. The strategy works for the first few weeks, only to stall around the third month or even later in case it is the first diet one undergoes.

This can be reversed by gradually increasing the calories ingested to raise the metabolism until the ideal caloric requirement is reached, taking a break from the diet, then starting a more moderate regimen again.

The best way to deal with the plateau would be to prevent it precisely with a gradual, balanced, nonrestrictive diet from the beginning, with a 10% deficit from the current requirement, and increase physical activity in intensity and frequency: this will result in slimming more slowly but less traumatically for the body, which will adapt to the new weight without objecting. If you want to intensify the weight loss, after 2-3 months, you can reach a 15% deficit in requirements by further increasing physical activity. After that, to maintain the weight you have achieved, gradually increase your energy intake (by 50 or 100 calories per week) until you reach your ideal requirement while continuing to exercise regularly and maintaining your healthy, balanced diet.

In addition to the overly direct dietary approach, the onset of the stall may also be influenced by other factors:

- The amount of lean mass contributes to raising the metabolism and accelerating slimming. Losing weight the wrong way, however, in addition to losing fat mass, also erodes lean mass, thus slowing down one's biological functions and weight loss.
- The subject's hormonal profile: since hormones regulate homeostasis, an imbalanced thyroid or steroid hormone profile can negatively affect metabolic parameters.
- In a miraculous way, the approach to dieting, especially if one expects to lose weight quickly and effortlessly, gives in to discouragement and temptation, constantly feeling deprived of the pleasures of food while not achieving results.
- Type and distribution of foods, which, while not unhealthy per se, may not be suitable for the specific phase of the diet or maybe maldistributed throughout the day. It is always a good idea to get advice from an expert nutritionist.
- Insufficient or unsuitable physical activity: for an overweight person, free body exercises, with weights or swimming, are more effective than, for example, jogging, which only risks straining the joints without giving real benefits.

The key to overcoming the stalemate, in general, is to understand where you are going wrong, to intervene early while also being ready to change strategy often depending on your body's reactions, but above all, to be patient and understand that weight loss cannot be a quick and automatic mechanism. Still, it must result from a profound and gradual change in your lifestyle.

Powerful questions

One of the things that helped me most in overcoming the stalemates was asking myself the following questions and actively seeking answers to improve my relationship with food, physical activity, and my new lifestyle. Let them inspire reflections in you, whatever they may be.

- *Am I consuming enough protein?*
- *Can I increase my physical activity?*
- *Am I drinking enough water?*
- *Are old habits creeping up on me?*

Do not forget that weight loss isn't a linear line going down at the same rate every week. On the contrary, it fluctuates and is affected by many factors. Consistency will be your number one ally when it comes down to your bariatric journey. The tool is not the start of a new diet. It's the beginning of a new lifestyle that requires a new mindset, personal growth, and support to get you closer to your goals.

Preventing food deficits

Even before surgery, bariatric surgery patients often have dietary deficiencies due to poor food choices and behaviors. What might these deficiencies be? They mainly concern vitamin B12, vitamin D, iron, and calcium. In addition, considering that patients may have other conditions besides obesity, it is necessary to make somewhat targeted and individual food choices: for example, for obese and hypertensive patients, it is good to always advise not to add table salt in the dishes as they are usually already salty, avoid certain types of foods, for example, canned meats and fish, bouillon cubes, pickles, and salted bread. In these cases, it is always good to minimize caffeine consumption.

Learning to read food labels and mineral waters is also very important.

Regarding the prevention of obese and diabetic patients, one of the strategies is not to consume fruit immediately after meals but to use it as a "meal-breaker," especially if you have not undergone a gastric bypass.

Another type of dietary choice concerns the obese person with dyslipidemia; in these cases, special attention should be paid to the diet without adding harmful fats (saturated fats), such as lard, cream, fatty meats, and sausages. In addition, it is necessary to be careful with foods that contain a lot of cholesterol, such as egg yolk, mushrooms, fats of animal origin; milk and its derivatives; some kinds of meat and fish, shellfish, and crustaceans.

CONCLUSION

Thank you for reaching the end of this cookbook. I hope you have found recipes that excite you give you the motivation to keep working on your GW. An air fryer is a great tool both for making healthy dishes and experimenting with the culinary art. My invitation is to make these recipes your own, modifying and integrating them in the way that best suits your taste and caloric requirements. I hope I have helped you realize that it is possible to follow the bariatric diet without giving up the flavors you like the most. Now it's up to you to continue the search for the perfect frying!

To thank you for reaching the end of my first cookbook, here is a picture of a puppy. He can't wait to see you smash your weight loss goals. Good luck!

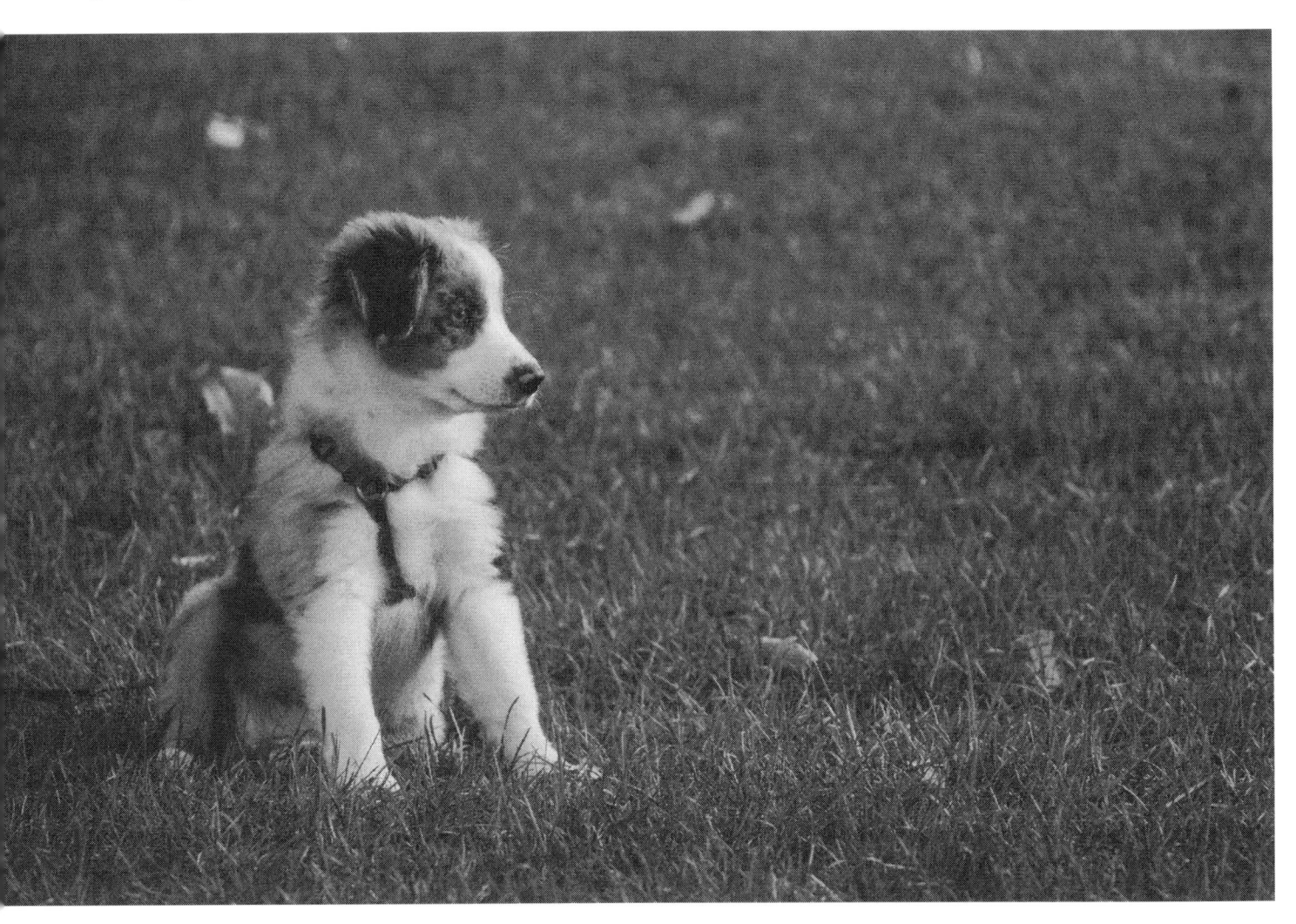

SHOPPING LIST

These are the ingredients required to cook all the recipes. Stock up your fridge and let's get started!

- agar agar
- almond flour
- almond milk
- almond milk
- almonds
- apple cider vinegar
- apples
- apricots
- asparagus
- avocado
- avocado oil
- bacon
- baking powder
- banana
- basil
- BBQ sauce
- beef steaks
- beef tenderloin
- bell peppers
- berry jam
- blueberries
- borlotti beans
- brandy
- bread
- breadcrumbs
- broccoli
- Brussel sprouts
- butter
- cabbage
- calamari
- cardamom
- carrots
- cashews
- cauliflowers
- cayenne
- cherry jam
- chicken breast
- chicken patties
- chili peppers
- chocolate
- chocolate chips
- cinnamon
- cocktail sauce
- cocoa powder
- coconut cream
- coconut milk
- coconut oil
- cod fillets
- coffee
- corn
- cornmeal
- cornstarch
- crab meat
- cream
- cream cheese spread
- cumin
- currant
- dates
- eggs
- flaked coconut
- flounder fillets
- garlic powder
- ginger
- ginger powder
- goji berries
- gorgonzola cheese
- greek yogurt
- ground pork
- ham
- hazelnuts
- honey
- hot sauce
- ketchup
- lamb chops
- lamb fillets
- leeks
- lemon juice
- lemons
- lentils
- liquid stevia
- macadamia nuts
- maple syrup
- marshmallows
- mascarpone cheese
- mayonnaise
- milk
- millet flour
- mozzarella cheese
- mustard
- nutmeg
- olive oil
- olives
- onion powder
- onions
- oranges
- oregano
- parmesan cheese
- parsley
- peaches
- peanut butter
- pears
- peas
- pecans
- pepper
- pineapple
- plums
- porchini mushrooms
- pork ribs
- potato starch
- potatoes
- pretzels
- puff pastry
- pumpkin
- raspberries
- ready-made tacos
- red wine
- rice
- rice flour
- roast beef
- rosemary
- rum
- salad
- salmon fillets
- salt
- sardines
- seed oil
- shallot
- smoked paprika
- sole fillets
- sour cream
- soy sauce
- spinach
- strawberries
- sugar-free orange juice
- sunflower oil
- sweet potatoes
- thyme
- tofu
- tomato paste
- tomatoes
- tortillas
- trout fillets
- tuna fillets
- turmeric
- vanilla extract
- vanilla ice cream
- vermouth
- vinegar
- walnuts
- whipped cream
- white wine
- zucchini

INDEX

Air fried biscuits 90
Almond cookies 90
Almond donuts 14
Almond sandwiches 74
Almonds and peanut butter balls 91
Apple and raisin pastries 91
Apple cake 15
Apple chips 92
Apple cinnamon pie 92
Apple pastries 93
Apple rolls 93
Apple treats 15
Apple-flavored bites 94
Avocado eggs 68
Avocado sticks 74
Bacon-wrapped avocado 75
Banana and chocolate brownies 16
Banana bread 16
Banana chips 17
Banana split 17
Beef and beans 50
Beef in red wine reduction 32
Beef kebab 50
Beef tacos 51
Beef tenderloin with butter 32
Bell pepper salad 68
Berry tacos 18
Blueberry pudding 75
Breaded sole 33
Breaded zucchini chips 76
Broccoli and cheese croquettes .. 33
Broccoli and mushroom omelet . 34
Broccoli and tofu risotto 34
Brussels sprouts with thyme and parsley 76

Butter and stevia pie 94
Butter cookies 18
Butter fried chicken 35
Butter salmon 35
Cake bites 94
Calamari rings with almonds 76
Calamari skewers in vermouth ... 51
Caramel and coconut cream 95
Cauliflower & cheese 35
Cauliflower and cheese gnocchi .. 77
Cauliflower balls 52
Cheese and bacon broccoli 77
Cheese cauliflower 78
Cheese fried zucchini 78
Cheese pork chops 52
Cheese sticks 78
Cheesecake treats 19
Cherry pie 95
Chicken breast 36
Chicken fajita with spicy potatoes 36
Chicken slices with peppers 52
Chicken wings 37
"Chipotle" steaks 50
Chocolate and peanut butter cookies 96
Chocolate balls 19
Chocolate cake 20
Chocolate chip cookies 20
Chocolate cream 21
Chocolate cupcake with chocolate cream 96
Chocolate cups 21
Chocolate mug cake 97
Chocolate pudding 21
Chocolate sufflè 97

Cinnamon cupcakes 79
Cinnamon pear chips 97
Cinnamon toast 22
Classic frankfurters 79
Classic schnitzel 53
Cocoa and almond bars 22
Coconut and honey apricots 98
Coconut and vanilla treats 79
Coconut-flavored brussels sprouts 53
Cod fillets with parmesan cheese 53
Coffee cake 22
Cookie doughnuts 23
Cordon bleu 37
Corn and tomato salad 68
Creamy salmon 38
Creamy zucchini and potatoes ... 69
Crispy apple chips 23
Crispy broccoli salad 69
Crunchy green beans 69
Cucumber and mozzarella wrap . 80
Currant and chocolate cupcakes 98
Danish cinnamon rolls 98
Deep-fried bananas with chocolate sauce 99
Easy biscuits 99
Eggs and tomatoes 70
Fish and chips 38
Fish tacos 54
Flounder fillets with parmesan cheese 54
Fried bananas 24
Fried cinnamon bananas 100
Fried chicken fillets 38
Fried peaches 24

Fried plantains 100
Fried sardines............................. 55
Garlic and spice chicken burger . 39
Garlic calamari............................ 55
Garlic pork tenderloins............... 39
German-style schnitzel............... 55
Gnocchi with parmesan cheese and cauliflower 56
Greek-style eggs......................... 80
Ham and bell pepper omelet 39
Hamburger and tzatziki 40
Hazelnut cake........................... 100
Healthy fries............................... 81
Herb crab cake 81
Herb lentils 70
Italian-style pork tenderloins 56
Kebab.. 40
Lamb burger 40
Lamb chops 57
Leek salad 70
Lemon butter cookies............... 101
Lemon lamb steaks 57
Lemon pie 82
Lentils and dates brownies........ 82
Meatballs.................................... 57
Meatloaf 41
Melted cheese cups 83
Mexican-style cheese sticks 83
Minced meat............................... 41
Mozzarella cheese cubes and paprika................................... 83
Mozzarella crostone with chicken and peppers 58
Mozzarella schnitzel................... 41
Mushroom, beef, and leek pie.... 42

Orange cookies........................... 25
Oregano clams 42
Oregano peppers....................... 71
Oriental-style asparagus............ 71
Oriental-style spiced lamb 58
Paprika and lemon grilled chicken 43
Paprika bacon cubes 58
Paprika pork ribs........................ 59
Parmesan trout.......................... 59
Peanut butter and jelly doughnuts 25
Peanut butter and marshmallow croissants.............................. 101
Pineapple sweets........................ 26
Pineapple yogurt sticks............ 102
Plain steak.................................. 60
Plum and currant cake............... 26
Poached apples.......................... 27
Porcini mushroom stake 43
Pork chops with 4 kinds of cheese 60
Pork ribs with parmesan cheese .60
Pork ribs..................................... 44
Puerto rican-style banana........... 84
Pumpkin cookies 27
Roast beef.................................. 44
Roasted nut mix......................... 84
Rum pancakes.......................... 102
Salmon fillets in walnut crust...... 61
Sausage and vegetable sandwich 44
Seasoned cod fillets 45
Seaweed chips 84
Sesame pork ribs........................ 62

Sesame-seasoned broccoli 85
Simple cookies 28
Smoked steaks 62
Snow-white cake........................ 28
Soft cake..................................... 85
Spice marinated chicken............ 63
Spiced pork steaks 63
Spicy bacon bites 86
Spicy hamburger 45
Spinach salad 71
Strawberry shortcakes.............. 103
Strawberry sweets..................... 86
Sweet potato croquettes 29
Sweet-and-sour pork steaks 64
Taco chips 87
Tangerine pudding..................... 87
Tasty salmon.............................. 45
Thyme and mushrooms meatloaf 64
Tofu with vegetables.................. 46
Trout with garlic and lemon 61
Tuna steak with red onions......... 65
Turkey and avocado burger 46
Turkey wings.............................. 46
Turmeric-orange marinated steak 65
Vanilla-cinnamon cookies......... 103
Vanilla cookies.......................... 103
Vanilla mug cake 104
Vanilla blueberry muffins........... 29
Vegetarian toast........................ 47
Western-style pork loin.............. 65
White wine chicken breast......... 47
Zucchini chips 87
Zucchini salad 72

Manufactured by Amazon.ca
Bolton, ON